The Pre-Psychoanalytic Writings of Sigmund Freud

edited by

Gertrudis Van de Vijver and Filip Geerardyn
University of Ghent, Belgium

Routledge
Taylor & Francis Group
LONDON AND NEW YORK

First published 2002 by Karnac Books Ltd.

Published 2018 by Routledge
2 Park Square, Milton Park, Abingdon, Oxon OX14 4RN
711 Third Avenue, New York, NY 10017, USA

Routledge is an imprint of the Taylor & Francis Group, an informa business

British Library Cataloguing in Publication Data
A C.I.P. for this book is available from the British Library

ISBN: 9781855752856 (pbk)

CONTENTS

4. Studies on Hysteria and The Neuro-Psychoses of Defence

5. The Project for a Scientific Psychology

6. Epistemological Issues: Materialism, Reductionism, and Evolutionism

A NOTE ON TEXTS

Where possible, quotations and references to Freud are given according to the *Standard Edition of the Complete Psychological Works of Sigmund Freud*, 24 volumes, translated and edited by James Strachey in collaboration with Anna Freud, assisted by Alix Strachey and Alan Tyson. London: The Hogarth Press and the Institute of Psycho-Analysis; New York: Norton, 1953-1974.

INTRODUCTION
THE ROOTS OF PSYCHOANALYSIS RECOVERED?

Gertrudis van de Vijver and Filip Geerardyn

This book was conceived in the wake of an international congress on Sigmund Freud's pre-analytic writings, which was held in May 1995 at the University of Ghent.[1] The congress attracted scholars from a vast variety of disciplines and schools. Their enthusiastic reactions, both during and after the conference, bore witness to the fact that this meeting was both important and unique.

The exploration of Freud's so-called 'pre-analytic' writings during the congress extended way beyond examination of purely historical data. The aim of this book, then, is to keep alive that spirit of research and co-operation. Firstly, we intend to transgress the rigid barriers erected between different disciplines, schools of thought and paradigms. Instead, we shall examine problems and possible solutions suggested by Freud's pre-analytic writings with an emphasis upon the respective *benefits* and inevitable losses that each approach yields, rather than concerning ourselves unduly with the polemics and presumptions of these approaches. Secondly, we aim at a cross-fertilisation of concepts and methods, by encouraging them to proliferate in entirely new fields. As Deleuze would have it, it is a matter of territorialising, de-territorialising and re-territorialising (Deleuze & Guattari 1991).

This *modus operandi* provides the most appropriate conditions under which to re-examine Freud's own intellectual daring and enthusiasm, in both theory and practice. It also seems to us the most suitable means of attempting to re-vitalise contemporary psychoanalytic theory and practice—by opening up avenues through *interrogation*, rather than seeking shelter within the confines of previously formulated answers.

But perhaps this course of action seems daunting when one considers the nature of the texts and ideas we shall be exploring. Freud's pre-analytic writings range over fields as diverse as histology, neurology, the psychophysics of cocaine, an engagement with French psychiatry, the philosophy of Franz Brentano and J.S. Mill, and his first, fledgling attempts at formulating a psychology inspired by his clinical experience of hysteria and the 'talking cure'.

The year 1900, the date of the publication of *The Interpretation of Dreams*, is traditionally, and quite arbitrarily, considered the starting-point for what have since become known as the 'psychoanalytical' writings. Whether or not 1900 is the correct date for the 'start' of psychoanalysis, it seems important to return to Freud's early writings in order to determine the relation of psychoanalysis to the other sciences. Indeed some of the sciences from which psychoanalysis arose—such as histology, neurology and psychophysics—boasted a much more respectable scientific status, and were never the subject of as many critical attacks. By relating psychoanalysis to its more 'respectable' roots, then, might it not be possible to demonstrate why and how it veered from its course, and then—perhaps—bring it back onto the 'secure road of a science'? But what is meant by 'the secure road of a science'? Although Kant described science in these terms,[2] it has now become apparent—more than two hundred years after the *Critique of Pure Reason*—that one must unrelentingly question this view. Is the 'secure road' today actually the same as that described by Kant? Interrogation of this kind must underlie any examination of the place occupied by psychoanalysis.

Freud himself displayed a continual commitment to *the spoken word*. Indeed, in this volume several authors illustrate the tacit choices made by Freud, and his empirical alertness regarding this matter, already manifest in his work on hypnosis (see Marone and Haimovich, below). It was on the basis of this line of approach—which he never abandoned—that Freud developed the analytic setting. The formulation of his psychological theory emerged, in effect, from within this setting and from the concentration on the spoken word which it entailed. Every science is confronted with the task of making more explicit the consequences of its methods and settings, and psychoanalysis is no exception to this rule.

Nevertheless, Freud's assumptions exhibit a striking peculiarity, in that, from the very beginning, he took the risk of *involving himself as a speaking being* within the setting. By doing this, he rendered the evaluation of his theory by external principles a much more complex task, because this approach results in the fact that one can never consider one's dreams, slips, mistakes, pathology—in short, *one's own speech*—as *external* to the one who is speaking.

In the course of this century, however, we have been confronted with variations on this problem in other fields—such as second order cybernetics (Van de Vijver 1996a), the theory of complex evolutionary systems (Matsuno, 1998; Matsuno & Salthe, 1995), and the immanentist interpretation in philosophy (Deleuze, 1993). In our view, it is along these lines that the 'secure road' of science should be rigorously reconsidered. What degree of certainty can be attributed to a science which does not succeed in describing situations in purely external terms, or—indeed—to a science which refuses to deny the dynamic and continually evolving nature of systems by freezing them in external descriptions?

Over the past century, numerous answers to these questions have emerged within the psychoanalytical field—for instance: the analysis of transference; identification; the status of speech as a means of externalisation; structuralism; topology and so on. Yet is it not the case that the various, conflicting points of view upon these, as well as the formation of a plethora of groups and schools of thought, point to the insufficiency of these solutions?

The aim of this book is not to pass judgement on the divergencies between these views, nor to tip the scales in favour of any one of them. Instead we aim to preserve the diverse and challenging character of Freud's pre-analytic writings. We do not cherish any belief in the potential of external arguments to shed light on the most recent developments in the field of psychoanalysis, and neither do we see any use in looking for an explanation of how, when and why things went 'wrong' in psychoanalysis, or in attempting to acquire a means of bringing psychoanalysis 'back into line'. Instead, we are more inclined to believe that the way ahead consists in adopting a radical approach to the notion of 'secure knowledge'. This shift implies a view of science which differs fundamentally from the classical, externalist approach. Only now, in the aftermath of the most recent developments in our understanding of self-organisation and complexity—the fallout from which is most perceptible in the fields of physics, biology, and cybernetics—does this message seem to stir up the general interest it deserves. Only now, in the context of an interdisciplinary approach, can these epistemological issues be taken up at the overlapping boundaries of the various disciplines concerned.

We do not intend to suggest that Freud, after his neurological and psychiatric beginnings, recoiled from consideration of his own project in relation to other sciences. Instead, it seems to us that relations between psychoanalysis and the other sciences came under considerable strain after the wider recognition of Freud's ideas. After the growth and intervention of the psychoanalytic institution, it seems, the original openness between psychoanalysis and the other sciences was lost.

This book, then, sets itself the task of 'listening to the tape' for a second time—not merely for the sake of hearing old music played over again, but to show how modern instruments can produce new sounds.

The organisation of this book

The reader will soon perceive the dominant assumption of this work: that *psychoanalysis possesses the status of a science*. Nevertheless, this does not silence other lines of approach, as will become clear in the course of successive chapters. Each section of this book focuses on a particular aspect of Freud's work, which we shall now introduce in more detail.

The beginnings in neurology and psychiatry

Only recently have Freud's neurological contributions attracted the attention they deserve. Scholars have now realised that Freud produced *outstanding* scientific achievements within neurology. In part, Freud himself was responsible for this lack of recognition; he was, after all, a leading advocate of the separation between his pre-analytic works and his psychoanalytic oeuvre. To give one instance: Freud acted against the advice of his collaborators in his decision not to include his monograph on aphasia in his *Gesammelte Schriften*. He must have had good reasons for this, and perhaps they included the fact that psychoanalysis—still a nascent discipline—needed to emancipate itself from medicine, particularly from psychiatry. Therefore, overt reference to the neurological roots of psychoanalysis was not considered opportune. Nevertheless, history has demonstrated that Freud's 'self-censorship' of his medical roots was of no avail. Despite his defence of 'lay analysis', psychoanalysis has tended to be viewed as the prerogative of physicians, or as an auxiliary discipline for psychiatrists.

Today, however, almost fifty years since the introduction of the large-scale use of psychopharmaceuticals, which sounded the deathknell of clinical psychiatry and announced the birth of biological psychiatry, the situation has altered greatly. In parts of Europe and South America psychoanalytic institutions—to a degree—actually succeeded in defending lay analysis. Here, at present, lay analysis appears to have achieved its independence. Elsewhere, in North America for instance, it is hoped that the ingrained prejudices against Freud's invention might one day be eliminated, perhaps by means of a fertile dialectic between psychoanalysis and the neurosciences (Solms 1996; Geerardyn & Quackelbeen 1996).

The papers collected in this first section, then, survey over two hundred articles dealing with Freud's neurological writings (Mark Solms). In addition to this, they pay homage to Freud as a psychiatrist (Hubert Van Hoorde), and offer a contribution to some present-day epistemological and clinical implications of Freud's work on aphasia (Filip Geerardyn).

'Coca'-Studies

When a major thinker has made a name for himself by laying the foundations of a new discipline, it is easy to understand how a tendency might arise to interpret the new work as being wholly unconnected to his earlier productions. Indeed, Freud's 'cocaine episode' seems—at first sight—a highly peculiar and uncharacteristic occurrence in his career.

Freud's interest was aroused by reports of the euphoric effects of cocaine. He ordered samples of it, in order to conduct experiments on himself, and immersed himself in the existing literature before publishing a substantial monograph on the coca plant. Freud praised the virtues of cocaine to his fiancée, and prescribed it to his friend von Fleischl—a morphine addict—which led to Fleischl's tragic death. The death of his friend, and the fact that it was not Freud but Konigstein (and, at a later date, Koller) who became famous for having put cocaine to use as a local anaesthetic, leads us to view this episode in Freud's life as shrouded in a mist of failure.

At least, this is what Freud himself seems to indicate (Freud 1900a: 169-76; 281-84). In his analysis of his dream of the botanical monograph he draws a parallel between his aborted ambition and the origin of his epistemological drive, yet he uses the dream to illustrate the discrepancy between latent and manifest content—that is, his own unwillingness (as the dreamer) to confront what actually happened during the cocaine episode. Paradoxically, however, his analysis of the dream actually sheds light on the originality of his work on cocaine. He was, after all, the first person to mention—albeit theoretically—that cocaine could function as an effective anaesthetic. Moreover, this passage reveals something about Freud's scientific ethics, since he freely gives credit to Koller as the person who put cocaine to a medical use.

The starting-point of Rik Loose and Pierre Eyguesier's contributions is Freud's fascination with cocaine as an 'ideal object'. This subjective dimension of Freud's work is supported by the historical research of Albrecht Hirschmüller. His meticulous reconstruction of the historical context of the cocaine episode enables reconsideration of the accepted version of these events. Did Freud lack critical judgement—as is sometimes argued? Did he accept far too unthinkingly the widespread belief in cocaine as an antidote to other addictions? Or does the fact that *he did not himself develop an addiction* reflect something significant—besides a certain degree of ego-strength?

Freud and philosophy

Freud attempted to ensure that psychoanalysis would not be conceived of and employed in the same way as a 'world-view', or as a purely philosophical conceptualisation of the human psyche. However, this aversion of Freud towards a world-view should not be mistaken for his general attitude towards philosophy.

His encounter with philosophers such as Franz Brentano demonstrates a wholly different perspective. Brentano introduced Freud to the works of Aristotle and J.S. Mill; he also encouraged Freud to translate a volume of J.S. Mill's collected works. A work by another philosopher—Wilhelm Jerusalem's *The Function of Judgement* (1895)—greatly inspired Freud's 'A Project for a Scientific Psychology' (Freud 1950a).

Even though Freud, in his writings, rarely alludes to the work of philosophers, his thought is permeated by the influence of Brentano, Mill, and Jerusalem. Indeed, the characteristic features of psychoanalysis were developed by Freud in a continuous—albeit tacit—dialogue with Aristotle's concept of the psyche (Geerardyn 1994). Freud drew on linguistic theory, influenced by the Anglo-Saxon tradition (Mill), and on a genetic conception of human language acquisition, which was by definition intersubjective (Jerusalem). In this volume, Aviva Cohen, Franz Kaltenbeck and Michael Molnar produce evidence which vividly reinforces the argument in favour of the influence of these thinkers upon Freud.

Studies on Hysteria *and the neuro-psychoses of defence*

Studies on Hysteria (Breuer & Freud 1895) is commonly acknowledged as a milestone in the genesis of psychoanalysis. However, its structure is not as linear as a first reading might suggest.

Studies on Hysteria begins with the 'Preliminary Communication' (Breuer & Freud 1893), in which both authors draw the readers attention to psychical defence mechanisms, in order to explain hysterical phenomena. However, this new approach is soon overshadowed by Breuer's theoretical chapter, which follows broadly physiological lines. It is Freud who brings the psychical to the foreground again, in his chapter on the therapy of hysteria. As is repeatedly demonstrated by the case histories included in the book, Freud focuses his attention upon the *speech* of the patient and 'the talking cure'. However, in his chapter on therapy, Freud does not convey a clear, univocal picture of the nature of the 'psychotherapy' or 'psychological analysis' which he uses. A re-reading of this text reveals that certain aspects of the *Studies*—for instance, the status of speech and memory, and the aim of the treatment—strongly resemble a Lacanian view of the psychoanalytic cure.

Aisling Campbell's paper, an examination of ethics in the field of psychiatry, draws on the lessons Freud learnt between the time of his studies under Charcot, and the publication of *Studies on Hysteria*. Katrien Libbrecht, meanwhile, examines the constitutional factor in the 'pre-analytic' explanation of neurosis, while Christfried Tögel sheds some new light on the case of Emmy von N., the fruit of his painstaking research in the archives of the Freud Museum.

The 'Project for a Scientific Psychology'

Freud's 'A Project for a Scientific Psychology' (Freud 1950a) is a key text. It was published posthumously, and appeared at the same time as Freud's correspondence with Fliess. The text employs a neurological frame of reference, and therefore provides direct evidence of Freud's thorough understanding of the neurology of his time. It also provides an insight into the clinical and psychological questions confronted by Freud in his attempt to treat cases of hysteria. Unlike the vast majority of Freud's pre-analytic works, this manuscript *has* received the attention it deserves.[3] However, this does not imply that a final agreement on the interpretation of this work has been reached. Some commentators still consider the 'Project' a failed attempt at a new understanding of the mind, undertaken by an author who oscillated uncertainly between neurology and psychology. Meanwhile, others have argued—by means of reductionist or evolutionist approaches—that the 'Project' contains the epistemological foundations of psychoanalysis.

The papers in this section of the book deal with both epistemological and clinical themes. David Smith, for instance, allocates a central place to the *materialism* of Freud's approach which—Smith argues—impelled Freud to forsake his Cartesian, dualistic conception of the mind-body problem. Smith pays special attention to the role of the Cartesian debate in Freud's elaboration of the unconscious and the advent of psychoanalysis.

Nathalie Charraud, Rivka Warshawsky and Helen Sheehan strike a different note. In the 'Project', Charraud identifies a unique understanding of signifiers which, in her view, liberates psychoanalysis from physiological reductionism, and accounts for some striking concordances between psychoanalysis, linguistics and mathematics. Warshawsky, in her paper, awards Freud's text the status of 'traumatic signifier'. As such, Freud was obliged to unceasingly revise the 'Project' throughout his career, in an unfinished attempt to circumscribe and define the psychoanalytic field.

Sheehan, meanwhile, argues that a psychoanalytic ethic is implied in Freud's notion of *'das Ding'* (the thing) which—in the 'Project'—arises from the first encounter with a fellow human being. Analysts who overlook this fact, she contends, doom their patients to perversion. Gertrudis Van de Vijver's contribution is to apply Freud's distinction between understanding and judging to a case dating from the beginning of the twentieth century. She analyses the notion of 'structure' in relation to identification, from both a pre-analytic and a contemporary perspective.

Epistemological topics: materialism, reductionism and evolutionism

The papers in this section of the book tie in most closely with our main argument—namely, that the challenging nature of Freud's pre-analytic texts lies in their potential to articulate a unique relationship between setting and theory. The authors in this section show how conception of the unconscious in dynamic and structural terms invites the accusation of 'reductionism'.

Saul Haimovich suggests that Freud's pre-analytic writings bear witness to an endeavour to combine an evolutionary conception of the psyche with a structural one. Freud's failure in this respect led him, in his metapsychological writings, to a 'psychological reductionism'. This was characterised by his abandonment of evolutionary-biological thinking in relation to the psyche. Haimovich urges us to restore evolutionary thinking to the field of psychoanalysis. The question then becomes how we can *combine* the structural and the evolutionary viewpoint.

Silvana Dalto explores how we should account for subjectivity, if we adhere to a materialistic view of psychical phenomena—as Freud so evidently does. This question appears to turn on the notion of how a system, when confronted with stimuli of various kinds, succeeds in unifying them and in achieving self-recognition from the incoming flux. Freud had already outlined an answer to this in the 'Project' but, in later texts, returned to it as the problem of 'identification'. Interestingly, Dalto's paper enables us to examine this problem from a strictly materialistic angle.

Fulvio Marone's contribution, drawing upon Freud's work on hypnosis, shows how the relationship between mind and body is obscured by methodological difficulties which make it impossible to draw an operational distinction between them. Freud confronts these problems head on, due to his refusal to conceive of the brain in accordance with the theory of localisation. Marone shows how Freud provides an explicit treatment of these issues in his work on aphasia, and in other writings.

Finally, Guy Trobas provides an account of Freud's evolution from an associationist conception of the unconscious to a structural view. This paper, drawing on the work of Lacan, illustrates the importance Freud attached to the idea that the psyche should be understood as a system which takes its shape according to its particular history.

In conclusion, it might seem an overt challenge to publish a volume on Freud's works, in the light of growing criticism of Freud within the fields of psychoanalysis, psychology, psychiatry, and the philosophy of science. What can be the significance or outcome of a book such as this, given a current climate which is highly laden with ideology, a climate in which 'killing Freud' prevails over reading him? Clearly, our aim is ambitious, and lies beyond any ideological claim. This reading of Freud's pre-analytic texts proposes, firstly, to introduce psychoanalysis to an alternative, research-driven, and interdisciplinary means of solving problems, and—secondly—to open up the possibility of a methodological shift in the sciences.

Whether the science of the new century will have incorporated Freud's message, or—as is heard more and more frequently—whether psychoanalysis will have been abandoned altogether, will depend upon the success of interdisciplinary initiatives, such as this one.

A note on the bibliography, and acknowledgements

We drew upon the *Freud-Bibliographie mit Werkkonkordanz* (Meyer-Palmedo & Fichtner 1989) for the bibliography of Freud's pre-analytic texts, and complemented it with translations in English, Dutch and Spanish. Some new references were added and corrections have made since it was first published.[4]

We would like to express our gratitude to all of those who helped us complete this bibliography, and to extend special thanks to: Albrecht Hirschmüller, Pat Jacops, Daniel Koren, Bert Lijsens, Lydia Marinelli, Michael Molnar, Inge Scholz-Strasser, Kathelijne Schoonjans, Mark Solms and Karin Temmerman. Finally, our thanks to everyone who reviewed or helped to translated the various contributions.

Notes

1 The organisers of the congress were F. Geerardyn, R. Loose, J. Quackelbeen, W.A. Szafran, and G. Van de Vijver. A substantially different volume of papers has appeared in French (Geerardyn & Van de Vijver 1998).

2 *'Den sicheren Gang (Weg) einer Wissenschaft'* (Kant 1982: 1).

3 See Buelens 1971; Hirschmüller 1989; Lacan 1978, 1986; Levin 1978; Pribram 1965; Pribram & Gill 1976; Sulloway 1979. For a more extensive list of references see Van de Vijver & Geerardyn 1992a.

4 See Van de Vijver & Geerardyn 1995: 107-152.

AN INTRODUCTION TO THE NEUROSCIENTIFIC WORKS OF SIGMUND FREUD

Mark Solms

Introduction

I am at the moment busy editing Freud's complete neuroscientific works for simultaneous publication in English and German, in four volumes. This is a very large body of work. Over a period of twenty-three years, between 1877 and 1900, Freud published more than two hundred neuroscientific titles, including forty original articles and six substantial monographs. However, a collected edition of these works—many of which are now very difficult to obtain, even in the original German—has never before been compiled. Only ten of these works have ever appeared in English translation, and even fewer in the other major languages. Most of them are not even listed in the *Standard Edition* bibliography of Freud's writings.[1]

When one considers the enormous impact of Freud's work on twentieth century science and culture, and the enduring fascination with his life and ideas, it is truly remarkable to discover that so large a portion of his scientific writings remains untranslated and inaccessible.

If it were true that Freud's pre-analytical writings were obscure and insignificant, then this might have been less remarkable. But Freud's neuroscientific works are anything but obscure and insignificant. They are of considerable interest, from both the neuroscientific and the psychoanalytic points of view. In almost every aspect of his work in the basic neurosciences, Freud made original contributions of note. This fact has long been acknowledged by neurological historians and Freud scholars alike. Also, those authors who have looked at these works in terms of their relevance to psychoanalysis have shown that they have the potential to enhance greatly our understanding of Freud's intellectual and scientific development. Psychoanalysis as a whole is, of course, inextricably interwoven with the life and work of Sigmund Freud. Therefore, we might reasonably expect that a greater familiarity with the genesis and early development of his ideas will improve and enrich our understanding of them. Indeed, it could even influence the future advancement of contemporary psychoanalysis by undoing accumulated distortions, omissions and misconceptions. Personally, I believe that a proper understanding of the origins of Freud's most basic concepts in the neurological sciences may also facilitate the difficult task which confronts those of us who are today attempting to reintegrate psychoanalysis with neuroscience. At the very least, greater familiarity with these works—as Freud himself wrote to Smith Ely Jelliffe in 1937—should 'have some influence on those who still like to believe that I pulled psychoanalysis out of my hat' (Burnham & McGuire 1983: 272).

In this chapter I shall introduce Freud's neuroscientific writings to the reader, in order to give an indication of their scope, their scientific merit, their historical importance, and—especially—their implications for psychoanalysis. However, I should state at the outset that because this is such a large body of work, I can only draw attention to a few selected themes. My aim is to provide a *broad overview* of Freud's neuroscientific works as a whole—that is, to convey something of the *context* within which the better-known works, such as 'the cocaine papers', 'the aphasia monograph', the 'Project', and the early writings on hysteria were situated.

I shall classify Freud's neuroscientific works into thematic groups, and provide comments on each of the major themes. There was a definite chronological progression in these themes, as Freud shifted his attention to ever more complex subjects—starting with elementary histological questions, and ending with the most complex problems of neuropsychology.

Histological and anatomical research

The first phase of Freud's neuroscientific activity—from 1877 to 1888—was devoted to histological and anatomical research. The first of these works was, in fact, not a piece of *neuro*scientific research at all. It was a study on the sexual anatomy of the eel. Its title in English translation is 'Observations on the Finer Structure of the Lobular Organs of the Eel, Described as Testicles'. The testicles of the eel had been a puzzling anatomical problem for centuries, because no-one could *find* them, and this had made it difficult to imagine how the species reproduced. In his study Freud dissected, in 400 specimens, an organ which seemed to be a likely candidate. However, in his conclusion, Freud declared that, to his great disappointment, he could not definitely decide whether the organ he dissected was the elusive testicle or not. In fact, as we now know with hindsight, Freud was actually the first anatomist to describe the initial *intersexuality* of this animal, but without recognising the significance of his findings. In being assigned this subject for his first piece of scientific work, Freud was made aware, from the very start of his career, of the central position that sexuality occupies in biology. Indeed, is it not remarkable that the discoverer of the castration complex began his career by searching, without success, for some 'missing' testicles?

The next four papers I shall single out represent the beginning of Freud's *neuro*scientific career.[2] These works were all concerned with the *histology of the nerve-cell*, the basic unit of all nervous tissue. The following quotation from Ernest Jones describes the broader context of this research:

> Together with the problem of the intimate structure of nervous elements... [there was the] question of whether the nervous system of the higher animals is composed of elements different from those of the lower animals, or whether both are built of the same units. This topic was highly controversial at that time. The philosophical and religious implications seemed to be very disturbing. Are the differences in the mind of lower and higher animals only a matter of degree in complication? Does the human mind differ from that of some mollusc—not basically, but correlative to the number of nerve cells in both and the complication of their respective fibres? Scientists were searching for the answers to such questions in the hope of gaining definite decisions—in one way or another—on the nature of man, the existence of God, and the aim of life. (Jones 1953: 51)

These early studies by Freud clearly belong to a vast and exciting field of research—and the contributions which Freud made to this field were quite fundamental. By studying the genetic migration and transformation of nerve cells in the spinal cord of a lowly fish called petromyzon, for instance, Freud showed that a continuous series of subtle changes linked the nervous system of the invertebrate with that of the vertebrate. Previously it was believed that a sharp anatomical division separated these two classes of animal. In other words, Freud discovered something of a 'missing link', and contributed to the great pool of data which finally established in the scientific community the conviction of the evolutionary continuity of all organisms. Freud also showed that traces of the phylogenetic migration and transformation of the nerve cells of this fish—over aeons—were still to be found in the spinal anatomy of the contemporary animal. Along the path originally traversed by the cells through evolution, Freud showed that some of the primitive forms of the cells had remained behind—fixated, as it were—in their phylogenetic development.

Freud's abiding commitment to *evolutionary theory*, and his belief in the persistence of primitive structures in the fully developed organism, can be traced back to these articles. Indeed, the connection is underscored by the fact that Freud *himself* referred to his research on the petromyzon in order to illustrate the concept of 'fixation' in his *Introductory Lectures on Psycho-Analysis*. He wrote:

> ...it is possible in the case of every particular sexual trend that some portions of it have stayed behind at earlier stages of its development, even though other portions may have reached their final goal. (Freud 1916-17: 340)

The second, and perhaps more important contribution arising from the series of early histological papers, was Freud's observation of the essential *morphological and physiological unity of the nerve cell and its axon*. This paved the way, in part, for the neurone theory. At the time that Freud conducted these researches—and it should be remembered that he was still a student at the time—the structural and functional relationship of nerve cells and nerve fibres was still highly controversial. Freud's observations led him to a novel point of view. In the summary to his 1884 paper he wrote:

> If we assume that the fibrils of the nerve fibre have the significance of isolated paths of conduction, then we would have to say that the pathways which in the nerve fibre are separate are confluent in the nerve cell: then *the nerve cell becomes the 'beginning' of all those nerve fibres anatomically connected with it*. But I should transgress the limitations I have imposed on this paper were I to assemble the facts supporting the reliability of this assumption. I do not know if the existing material suffices to decide this important problem. If this assumption could be established it would take us a good step further in the physiology of the nerve elements: we could imagine that the a stimulus of a certain strength might break down the isolated fibrils so that *the nerve as a unit*

> *conducts the excitation*, and so on. (Jones 1953: 54, emphasis added)

These are the basic elements of the neurone theory, but the way in which Freud presented his findings was far too vague and reserved for him to deserve credit for the discovery of the neurone. A full seven years would pass before Waldeyer and Cajal formally proclaimed its existence.

Once again, then, Freud had made observations of the greatest theoretical importance without actually allowing himself to realise it. In fact Brazier (1959), in her standard work on the history of neurophysiology, also credited Freud with having adumbrated Sherrington's synapse concept—which completed our modern picture of the neurone. In a more recent monograph by Gordon Shepherd (1991), an entire chapter is devoted to a discussion of Freud's contribution to the theory.

Today, of course, the neurone doctrine is no longer even described as a 'doctrine'; it is the unquestioned cornerstone, the basic building-block, of all neuroanatomical and neurophysiological theory. It therefore seems ironic that years later, when Freud turned his scientific attention to the problems of psychology, he was roundly accused of leaping too quickly from observation to theory. The fact that the young Freud did not draw the necessary conclusions from these crucial observations, it seems to me, either contradicts the accusation that he was inclined to jump too quickly from observation to theory, or else it explains why he was later inclined to do so!

Two decades after these histological researches, Freud built an elaborate model of the mind around the concept of the neurone in his 1895 'A Project for a Scientific Psychology' (1950a). Even so, there is no hint in this text of the idea—which must by then have been clear to him—that he could have secured for himself a seminal role in the development of that concept.[3]

Next, I shall focus upon a small set of *methodological* papers which Freud published during this phase. In the first of these papers, entitled—in English translation—'Note on a Method for the Anatomical Preparation of the Nervous System' (1879), Freud reported a new method of separating nervous tissue from the surrounding muscle and bone. In a subsequent article he described a new technique for staining nerve cells, which had enabled him to see them more clearly under the microscope (1884e). To his great disappointment, however, the technique was never widely accepted. It seems that it was a difficult and fragile method—temperamental, even. In Freud's hands it yielded a wealth of observations and discoveries, but few of his colleagues had the sensitivity and patience to achieve comparable results. It could be said that a similar fate awaited the psychoanalytic method.

Freud had also described a new technique in one of the histological papers concerned with the structure of the nerve fibres and cells of the river crayfish. While studying the nerve cells of this animal, Freud became dissatisfied with the standard technique of observing dead cells under the microscope. Instead he employed a new technique which enabled him to observe the internal workings of the living cell. Suddenly, a host of structures and processes which had previously been invisible appeared before him. It is to this discovery, perhaps, that we may trace Freud's later awareness of the effects that the act of observation has upon the object being observed. Herein, too, may lie the seeds of his later rejection of artificial laboratory methods, in favour of natural observation of the living subject in a controlled setting.

In any event, with all of these new methods, which greatly facilitated the anatomical discoveries I shall now describe, Freud grasped the fact—so important for his later psychological work—that progress in science almost always flows from new methods of observation.

In his next three anatomical papers Freud painstakingly mapped out unknown territories in two small, densely packed, and extremely intricate parts of the brainstem, known as the medulla oblongata and the pons.[4] In the course of these works, Freud progressed from the spinal cord upwards to the brain itself, and also from the individual nerve cell to groups or constellations of cells. Simultaneously he shifted from the animal to the human nervous system.

In these studies Freud demonstrated the links between the posterior spinal columns and the cerebellum, and he traced the termination and connections of the acoustic nerve in the medulla. Overall, these were valuable contributions to basic neuroanatomy. He also formulated the theory that the sensory cranial nerve nuclei are homologous with the posterior nerve roots of the cord. He thus brought simple order to a once chaotic and opaque region of the brain. These days, medical students simply learn by rote the anatomy of the cranial nerves, from textbooks available in their local bookshop. It is hard to imagine that, barely one hundred years ago, pioneers such as Freud laboriously developed new microscopic staining techniques, in order to visualise, identify and classify these nerves within the impenetrable maze of cells and fibres which makes up this highly complex part of the body.

When considered from the vantage-point of his later work, Freud's methodology in his work on the human brainstem was especially interesting. Instead of attempting to map out directly the masses of fibre-paths, Freud studied the much simpler patterns which can be more easily observed in the foetal and infantile brain. Then, methodically, he traced the later developments across increasingly more mature specimens. So here too, the genetic (or developmental) point of view is paramount, and the evolutionary approach again conspicuous in Freud's conceptualisation of his results.[5]

Freud's last article on pure anatomy was published in 1888, and was entitled simply 'The Brain' (1888c). It was a summary of the state of the art in nineteenth century brain anatomy and physiology. This article is important because, apart from the 1895 'Project', it is the only place in which Freud ever published his views on the structure and function of the human brain as a whole.[6]

However, I should mention that this article cannot be attributed to Freud with absolute certainty, because it was unsigned—although internal evidence demonstrates beyond any reasonable doubt that at least the anatomical half of the article was written by him. Although written in the form of a reference work or encyclopaedia entry, Freud used this article as an opportunity to develop an entirely new theory of human brain anatomy, replacing the established anatomical theory of his esteemed teacher Theodor Meynert. Almost none of Meynert's anatomical teachings have endured—they are today mockingly referred to as 'brain mythology'—whereas Freud's alternative theory, by contrast, is broadly compatible with modern neuroanatomical views. Freud went on to develop this anatomical model further, in his 1891 monograph 'On Aphasia' (1953), which is examined in more detail below. Freud also wrote a manuscript on his anatomical model of the brain, in 1886. Although it was never published, a copy survives in the Library of Congress, Washington.

The cocaine episode

Whilst Freud was completing his anatomical studies, he published a series of six articles on the alkaloid known as cocaine. These pioneering and controversial studies are discussed elsewhere in this volume, therefore I will comment only upon some of the bare facts of Freud's work in this area.

The first paper, entitled simply 'On Coca' (1884b), is the major work in this series. It is, as Jones claims, a literary masterpiece,

> couched in Freud's best style, with all his characteristic liveliness, simplicity and distinction, features for which he had little scope in describing the nerves of the crayfish or the fibres of the medulla. (Jones 1953: 90)

The paper sets out to summarise everything that was known about this obscure drug from South America. The most interesting section, however, contains a number of observations by Freud concerning the effects of cocaine upon himself. He writes of 'an exhilaration and lasting euphoria... an increase of self-control... and vitality and capacity for work... without any of the unpleasant after-effects brought about by alcohol', yet 'absolutely no craving for the further use of cocaine appears even after repeated taking of the drug' (Jones 1953: 91). Freud goes on to describe cocaine's possible therapeutic usefulness in the treatment of, amongst other things, neurasthenia, melancholia and morphine addiction, and formulates an exacting theory of its neurochemical action. These suggestions and formulations establish Freud—as Robert Byck (1974) has acknowledged—as one of the founders of psychopharmacology.

In the final, fateful paragraph of this monograph, Freud added the following words:

> The capacity of cocaine to anaesthetise cutaneous and mucous membranes suggests a possible future use—and some additional applications of cocaine based on this anaesthetic property are likely to be developed in the near future. (Jones 1953: 91)

Indeed, they were. But it was Carl Koller, not Freud, who developed them—to great acclaim. Thus Freud, once again, narrowly missed out on fame at an early age. As he later wrote in his *Interpretation of Dreams*: 'I had not been thorough enough to pursue the matter further' (Freud 1900a: 170). The other therapeutic promises Freud had seen in the drug came to nothing. Freud was left reproaching himself with having hastened the death of a dear friend, by inculcating in him a severe cocaine addiction. Indeed, he was accused by some of his colleagues of having introduced to the world 'the third scourge of humanity'—the other two being alcohol and morphine. The complex and ambivalent feelings aroused in Freud by the whole episode are chronicled in his celebrated dreams of 'the botanical monograph' and 'Irma's injection'. Nevertheless, there can be no doubt that in the sentences from the final paragraph of the work, which I quoted above, Freud at least predicted the local anaesthetic properties of cocaine.

Most of Freud's other cocaine papers are simply summaries or elaborations of the first work.[7] Only two of them will receive mention here. The 1885 paper, entitled 'Contribution to Knowledge of the Effects of Cocaine' (1885b), represents the first and only experimental study that Freud ever published. I agree with those who have argued that it was a bad and poorly-controlled experiment. Freud's talents clearly did not lie in this direction—which is interesting, in view of his later remarks about the uselessness of the experimental method in psychology.

The last paper in the cocaine series, 'Craving for and Fear of Cocaine' (1887), was Freud's belated rejoinder to all of the criticisms levelled against him by his colleagues, when the tide of medical opinion turned against the drug. This, too, is a disappointing work, full of excuses and rationalisations. In it Freud constructs an elaborate and unconvincing theory of the lability of the cerebral blood vessels to account for the unpredictable action of cocaine, and he lays the blame for all its ill-effects on the innocent hypodermic needle. Here Freud's guilt-ridden dream of 'Irma's injection' again comes to mind.

It is interesting to note, in these studies, Freud's first published *self-observations*, which would culminate in the catalogue of self-revelation that he published in *The Interpretation of Dreams*. This serves to remind us that introspection and self-experiment were common scientific paradigms in the late nineteenth century. The significance of this fact for the development of the psychoanalytic method is seldom recognised.

A strong case can be made for the view that Freud's experience of the effects of cocaine upon sexuality and general arousal must have been an important source for his later libido theory, and perhaps for the economic point of view in general. Consider for example the following passage from the *Three Essays on the Theory of Sexuality*:

> It must suffice us to hold firmly to what is essential in this view of the sexual process: the assumption that substances of a peculiar kind arise from the sexual metabolism. For this apparently arbitrary supposition is supported by a fact which has received

> little attention but deserves the closest consideration. The neuroses, which can be derived only from disturbances of sexual life, show the greatest clinical similarity to the phenomena of intoxication and abstinence that arise from the habitual use of toxic, pleasure-producing substances (alkaloids). (Freud 1905c: 215-216)

As we can see, Freud's often-expressed opinion that the libido theory would someday be grounded upon a chemical substratum can also, apparently, be traced back to the experiences that he reported in the early cocaine studies.

Clinical neurology

During the cocaine period Freud gradually moved away from histology and anatomy, towards the problems of clinical neurology. This is the next major theme in Freud's neuroscientific writings. With his writings on these problems Freud graduated fully from controlled laboratory preparations to living, clinical cases. It is extremely unusual, especially today, for an individual scientist to be gifted both in the techniques of the anatomical laboratory and the hospital clinic, but evidently Freud was such a person.

Freud's first three articles in this field were all single-case studies.[8] The American neurologist Jelliffe has described them as 'models of good neurological deduction' (Jelliffe 1937: 696). Freud was an extremely capable neurologist, and he is reputed to have been able to localise the site of a brain lesion so accurately—on the basis of the patient's presentation during life—that the pathological anatomist had nothing to add to Freud's clinical formulations in the autopsy report. The fame of his diagnostic skills brought him a flurry of foreign graduate students. However, Freud himself spoke disparagingly of this talent. He later remarked that focal neurological diagnostics was 'a silly game of permutations' (Bernfeld 1951: 214).

It was after writing these early case-studies that Freud undertook his period of study under Charcot, at the Salpêtrière in Paris. During this period (between 1885 and 1886) Freud moved from being under the direct, personal influence of some of the leading figures of the German school of neurology, to being under the direct personal influence of Charcot. This shift had a decisive influence on his thinking. This was not so much a shift away from neurology towards psychology—as is usually suggested—but rather a shift away from the mechanistic anatomical explanations of clinical syndromes which was so characteristic of the neurology of Freud's German teachers. Instead, he moved towards the rich clinical descriptions which were characteristic of the French school of neurology under Charcot. The following quotation—from Freud—graphically illustrates the difference between these two schools:

> Charcot... never tired of defending the rights of purely clinical work, which consists in seeing and ordering things, against the encroachments of theoretical medicine. On one occasion there was a small group of us, all students from abroad, who, brought up on German academic physiology, were trying his patience with our doubts about his clinical innovations. `But that can't be true,' one of us objected, `it contradicts the Young-Helmholtz theory [of colour vision].' He did not reply `So much the worse for the theory, clinical facts come first' or words to that effect; but he did say something which made a great impression on us... [He said: `Theory is good; but it doesn't prevent things from existing'.] (Freud 1893d: 13)

This was one of Freud's favourite anecdotes. It reminds one of the lines spoken by Mephistopheles in Goethe's *Faust* (part 1, scene 4), which Freud also cited (more than once) with approval: 'Grey, dear friend, is all theory,/ And green alone Life's eternal tree'.

When Freud returned to Vienna, he declared himself to be an enthusiastic disciple of Charcot, and henceforward abandoned the 'grey' of anatomical theory in favour of the 'green' of clinical life. What is of fundamental importance here, I think, is the fact that Freud displayed the same new-found respect for careful clinical observation, description and classification in both his neurological and his psychological publications from this period, and the same aversion to ad hoc physiological and anatomical explanation of the clinical symptoms, regardless of whether the condition in question was functional or organic.

I agree with the paediatric neurologist Pasquale Accardo, who wrote the following words, not about Freud's psychological writings, but about his neurological research following his period of study under Charcot:

> ...what can only be called a 'conversion' from mechanistic physiology to clinical medicine occurred during Freud's travelling fellowship to the Salpêtrière (1885 to 1886), when he fell under the influence of the great neurologist, Charcot... Charcot breathed life into his previously sterile clinical expertise. (Accardo 1982: 452)

This underlying shift in Freud's neuroscientific allegiances must surely have been decisive for the breakthrough into psychoanalysis. By shifting his attention to the subjects of hysteria and neurasthenia from 1886 onwards, Freud was not shifting his attention away from neurology. Hysteria and neurasthenia were very much problems of neurology in the late nineteenth century. Freud continued to publish literally hundreds of works on a wide range of neuroscientific topics together with his early writings on hysteria and other neuroses. There was nothing unusual about that; the neuroses were generally conceptualised as nothing other than functional disturbances of the nervous system—by Freud as well as by everybody else. What distinguished these neurotic disorders from other nervous diseases was the fact that no anatomical lesion could be found at autopsy. This is why Freud's shift to the French (clinical-descriptive) school of neurology, and away from the German (anatomical-explanatory) school, paved the way for the breakthrough into psychoanalysis. For how could one elucidate the anatomical mechanism of a disorder in which no anatomical disease process could be demonstrated by the pathologist? Here the French school had a decisive advantage. Whereas Freud's German teachers could only construct speculative anatomical models, or reject the topic out of hand as being unsuitable for scientific study, the French neurologists could treat the neuroses as—to quote Freud—'just another topic in neuropathology' (Freud 1893d: 20). They could study the neuroses in precisely the same way as they had studied every other nervous disorder, namely, by systematically describing and defining its clinical manifestations, in order to arrive at a deeper understanding of its essential nature. This was clearly the only empirical way to proceed with the neuroses at that time. And from there it was only a small step from *looking* at the patient (as Charcot did) to *listening* to her (which Freud did). In turn, this approach led to the fundamental clinical observations which laid the foundations of psychoanalysis.

However, it should be remembered that Freud only gradually developed his newly-acquired skills as a truly clinical researcher when he returned to Vienna, as he continued to publish in neurological journals. Considering his publications from this period, I am going to ignore (for present purposes) the papers on hysteria and related topics. I would like, instead, to trace the progression of his papers on organic neurological diseases, in order to demonstrate my point that this was far from being an exhausted field of interest for Freud, and also to show that the actual shift to psychology came quite a few years later.

In his 1885 paper, 'A Case of Muscular Atrophy with Widespread Disturbances of Sensibility' (1885d), Freud became only the second neurologist ever to describe a case of *syringomyelia*. In a subsequent paper, 'Acute Multiple Neuritis of the Spinal and Cranial Nerves' (1886a) he became the first Viennese physician to diagnose the condition. It is an excruciatingly painful disease, and it is interesting to read Freud's detached clinical account of his patient's nightmarish decline and death. It is a very far cry from the sympathetic studies of the subjective experiences of his hysterical patients, which he would publish just a few years later, after his return from Paris.

Simultaneously, throughout this period, Freud was also publishing an enormous number of reviews of the contemporary neuroscientific literature. Most of these reviews have only recently been discovered—by Gerhard Fichtner. These short works demonstrate a remarkable mastery of the international neuroscientific literature—German, English, French and Italian—on every conceivable topic. It is fascinating to read Freud's critical appraisals of the works of some of his contemporaries—like Dejerine, Sachs, Bechterew and Babinski—who became major figures in the history of neurology.

Finally, the full impact of Charcot's influence emerged in a paper entitled 'On Hemianopia in Earliest Childhood' (1888a). It was the first report on a visual symptom which sometimes occurs in young children, the existence of which—today—is firmly established.

This was Freud's first publication in the new field of paediatric neurology—yet another branch of neurological science in which he was an acknowledged pioneer. It also marked the next phase in his scientific development.

Freud conducted his clinical research in this field as Director of the Neurological Department of the Institute for Children's Diseases in Vienna, during the last decade of the century. During this period Freud published a series of major works on the subject of cerebral palsy—that is, of movement disorders caused by brain damage near the beginning of life. These were truly monumental works which brought Freud international fame as the world's leading authority on the subject. Later, all sorts of criticisms were made about Freud having constructed a developmental theory on the basis of observations made on adults. Evidently, it was not appreciated just how much direct experience of working with sick children Freud actually had—although it is, of course, true that these were not psychoanalytical observations. Nevertheless, an investigation of the mental status of the child was a routine part of the clinical work in Freud's paediatric neurology department.

Freud wrote three long monographs on cerebral palsy in children. The first of these, co-written with his life-long friend Oscar Rie (who appears in the dream of Irma's injection as 'my friend Otto') was published in 1891 (Freud & Rie 1891). It examines the unilateral paralyses of children from every conceivable point of view. It is 220 pages long, includes a bibliography of 180 titles, and details Freud's personal observations on thirty-five cases. A second monograph (1893a) appeared as a supplement to the former, and dealt with the bilateral paralyses of children. It reports Freud's observations on a further fifty-three clinical cases. The third monograph (1897a) covers the combined ground of the previous two—in other words, *all* the movement disorders of childhood. It is an absolutely exhaustive and comprehensive treatise, a full 327 pages long. The bibliography alone spans fifteen pages.

These three monographs were interspersed by a long series of shorter writings on cerebral palsy, most of which were merely summaries of the big works, or reviews of writings by others. A short paper on childhood enuresis, published in 1893, is worthy of mention in the present context (1893b). It expounds an entirely neurological conception of the complaint.

I am mindful of what might seem the uncritical praise I am lavishing on Freud's neurological works. However, the following quotation, from a non-analyst, provides an equally positive assessment of Freud's reputation in the field of paediatric neurology:

> The student of the movement disorders of children... cannot fail to be impressed by the sheer magnitude, as well as the clinical acumen, of Freud's investigations into the cerebral palsies of childhood. The developmental perspective that he pioneered has only recently been fully appreciated... [He produced] some of the most masterly and exhaustive treatises to date on the cerebral

> paralyses of children. In addition to the typically Germanic erudition with which he reviewed the world literature, Freud reported many perceptive clinical observations. For example, he was the first to describe homonymous hemianopia in [infantile] hemiplegia. He noted the ease with which hemiplegia could be diagnosed simply by placing the child on a flat surface, and he described the occurrence of simultaneous or mirror movements—the involuntary participation of a paralysed limb in the intentional movements of the uninvolved side. He originated a typology of classic postures—constrained postures and unintentionally assumed resting poses representing structures of least resistance. Freud proposed a considerably expanded definition of cerebral palsy when he hypothesised the existence of numerous attenuated and benign forms, paradoxical cases of 'cerebral palsy without paralysis'. Freud's contribution to the classification of cerebral palsy was revolutionary. A neuropathologist by training, he was nevertheless forced to conclude that the optimal nosology was purely clinical, as the neuropathologic findings bore little or no consistent relationship to the clinical picture. When neuroanatomic localisation proved an unobtainable goal, Freud had to search elsewhere for an explanation of the observed symptoms. His solution to this problem was developmental... almost all observed clinical idiosyncrasies 'can be traced back to the fact that the disease affects an incompletely developed brain and a growing organism' (Freud 1968: 109). Thus, chorea and athetosis, ataxia and spasticity, were seen as ontogenetic stages in normal infants, transient infantile movement patterns that would later be suppressed by the evolution of higher centres. Freud's classification imposed a degree of order on half a century of chaos, and his correlations between clinical observation and neuropathology expressed concepts that are still in the vanguard of critical thinking about cerebral palsy today. (Accardo 1982: 452-453)

The relationship of normality to pathology is obviously fundamental to psychoanalysis—one need only think about the *Three Essays on the Theory of Sexuality* to see how directly Freud carried these ideas over into psychology. Here we can also clearly recognise the shift that I emphasised earlier, away from the anatomical-explanatory tradition of the German neurologists, to the clinical-descriptive approach of the

French school of Charcot. Also apparent is the transition from anatomical localisationism, to the dynamic, functional and developmental approach which established the conceptual scaffolding for psychoanalysis. Schott (1981) has discussed these issues in detail, in his important article on Freud's cerebral palsy monograph.

My reason for emphasising so strongly the importance of these works is that—I believe—they demonstrate the intimate bond between psychoanalysis and clinical medicine. I think this has important implications for modern researchers, who are attempting to re-integrate psychoanalysis with neurological science, and with mainstream science in general, but on the basis of precisely the sort of reductive methods that Freud rejected more than one hundred years ago. History has a lot to teach us in this regard, especially in an age in which experimental and laboratory techniques are so idealised, and the beauty and complexity of the 'green tree of life', to which Goethe referred, is so neglected. I think it is no exaggeration to say that today psychoanalysis stands as one of the last outposts of the great clinical traditions of internal medicine, and it would be to the detriment of science as a whole if we were to abandon that allegiance.

Neuropsychology

From 1891, we enter the last phase in Freud's neuroscientific research. We see him shifting away from physical neurology, towards neuropsychology, and then gradually into psychoanalysis. Freud's two major neuropsychological works were his monograph *On Aphasia* (1953), and his 'A Project for a Scientific Psychology' (1950a). As these works are explored in depth elsewhere in this volume, I will limit myself to a few scattered remarks.

The monograph on aphasia is, in my view, Freud's neurological *magnum opus*—it is an undisputed work of genius, which continues to be cited to this day in standard neuropsychological and aphasiological textbooks (Freud 1953). Walther Riese (1958), one of the world's foremost neurological historians, called it 'a rare and brilliant piece of medical thought' (Riese 1958: 289).

I will mention just a few of the innovations that it introduced. The fundamental argument of the work was that language, being a psychological organisation, cannot be mapped in a crude one-to-one fashion onto the anatomy of the brain, as there is no direct correlation between the elementary concepts of neurology and those of psychology. Starting from this premise, Freud introduced a new conceptualisation of the nature of aphasic disorder. On the basis of this conceptualisation, Freud is sometimes credited with having been the first to advocate a truly psychological study of neurologically impaired patients, and therefore of having been one of the founders of modern neuropsychology.

In his book, Freud, by carefully reasoned argument, integrating his clinical and anatomical knowledge, demolished the orthodox doctrine of narrow localisationism and exposed the fundamental methodological flaws in nineteenth century clinico-anatomical correlation. He replaced it with the dynamic, functionalist conception which flourished in the middle decades of the present century, and inspired some outstanding modern neurologists, such as A.R. Luria. The functionalist model of cognition which Freud developed in this monograph is also highly compatible with the connectionist models which are currently so fashionable. It was also in this book that Freud introduced the powerful 'agnosia' concept, which has had an enormous impact on all subsequent conceptions of higher cortical dysfunction. He also adumbrated von Monakow's 'diaschisis' concept, questioned the clinical validity of 'conduction aphasia' (which is still controversial today), and introduced many other modern notions too numerous to mention here. The list is almost endless. In many respects, this book represented a turning-point in modern theoretical neuroscience.

But this book is not only a neurological classic; it also represents Freud's first foray into the field of psychology. The anatomical model Freud developed in his aphasia monograph, and the re-conceptualisation of the notion of cerebral localisation that went along with it, re-appears in his 'Some Points for a Comparative Study of Organic and Hysterical Motor Paralyses' (1893c). It re-emerges in Letter 112 of the Fliess correspondence, and in his subsequent writings on the psychical mechanism of hysteria. Indeed, here it forms the conceptual bedrock of his assertion that hysterical symptoms have nothing to do with the anatomy of the brain, and that they arise instead from what he called 'lesions of ideas'. It is therefore unsurprising that an understanding of Freud's aphasia monograph is crucial for an understanding of all his later psychological models. It was perhaps for this very reason that the editors of the original *Gesammelte Schriften* wanted to include it with his collected psychological works. It was Freud himself who prevented this. For whatever reason, he seemed to want to maintain a sharp division between the two periods of his working life. Even so, Strachey still felt it necessary to append two lengthy extracts from this monograph to his translation of Freud's metapsychological essay, 'The Unconscious'.[9]

Finally, then, we arrive at his 'A Project for a Scientific Psychology' (1950a), another indisputable work of genius, which is legitimately considered a seminal psychoanalytic text. All the fundamentals of Freud's later topographic, dynamic and economic models were elaborated here for the first time. But the 'Project' is also very interesting from a neuroscientific point of view. Pribram and Gill (1976) argue that the 'Project' represents a sophisticated cognitive neuropsychological theory, even by today's standards. However, this assessment was made twenty years ago.

Before ending this survey of Freud's neuroscientific writings, it should be mentioned that Freud continued to publish numerous short articles, medical encyclopaedia entries, and many, many reviews, on a wide range of neurological topics, right up until 1900. I will draw attention to only two of them.

One is an article on amnesia which was published in 1893 (Freud 1893-94). This previously unknown work, which was only recently discovered, contains an extremely interesting theory of the forgetting of dreams. In fact, the article seems to have more to say about dreams than about amnesia. It seems, therefore, to be Freud's first published work on the subject of dreaming. The theory of the forgetting of dreams expounded in this article is almost identical with the 'state-dependent' theory of our own times. This is a theory which—ironically—is now being cited as an alternative to the views on forgetting which Freud developed later, in the *Interpretation of Dreams* and *The Psychopathology of Everyday Life.*

The second article I shall mention is a review of an essay on migraine by Möbius, which is quite interesting from the psychoanalytical point of view, and also for the reason that Freud describes his own personal experiences of migraine in it (Freud 1895).[10]

It seems to me that many of the works included in the *Standard Edition* deserve also to be included among Freud's neuroscientific papers. And I am referring not only to the 'Project'. If one considers Freud's earliest writings on hysteria and neurasthenia—which were as much problems of neurology at the end of the nineteenth century as they were of psychiatry—it will be seen that these works are methodologically and theoretically continuous with Freud's largely nosological writings on physical neurological topics from the same period.

Ironically, because of the sharp division that has traditionally been drawn between Freud's neurological and psychological writings, some of Freud's early so-called psychological writings have not received the attention from neurological historians that they deserve. Here I will mention again Freud's comparative study of organic and hysterical paralysis (Freud 1893c). This is an unrecognised work of some considerable neurological importance. Almost every point which Freud makes in that article on the differential diagnosis of neurogenic and psychogenic paralyses is now generally accepted clinical wisdom, and is taken absolutely for granted in neurological diagnosis. Indeed, as with so many of Freud's early works, I was amazed to discover that these ideas originated from him, and then surprised that he did not receive the credit for them.

Notes

[1] Where explicit reference is made to these works, the original German publications are given in the bibliography.

[2] I am referring to the works listed in the bibliography as 1877 (which was completed after the study on the eel, but published before it), 1878, 1882 and 1884c (which was in fact written in 1882).

[3] Incidentally, in the four histological studies under consideration here, Freud also provided an early account of microtubule research—before microtubules had even been discovered—and he unwittingly became the first to report the phenomenon of nuclear rotation of neurones in culture (Triarho & del Cerro 1985).

[4] These papers are listed as 1885e ('Contribution to knowledge of the inter-olivary layer'); 1886b ('On the relationship of the restiform body to the posterior column nucleus, with observations on two fields of the oblongata'); and 1886c ('On the origin of the nervus acusticus').

[5] Incidentally, the method that Freud used here was first pioneered by Paul Flechsig, who later featured in Freud's psychoanalytic writings as the subject of Judge Schreber's paranoid delusions.

[6] A comparison of these two works—the 1888 article on the brain and the 1895 'Project'—reveals many interesting facts, which I have discussed in a book that I published on this article in 1990, and therefore will not repeat here (see Solms & Saling, 1990).

[7] These are listed in the bibliography as 1884d, 1885a, 1885b, 1885c and 1887.

[8] These are listed in the appendix as, firstly, 1884a ('A Case of Brain Haemorrhage with Indirect Basal Focal Symptoms'); secondly, 1885d ('A Case of Muscular Atrophy with Widespread Disturbances of Sensibility [Syringomyelia]'); and, thirdly, 1886a ('Acute Multiple Neuritis of the Spinal and Cranial Nerves').

[9] It is not well known that Freud also published two shorter works on the subject of aphasia. In view of the importance of this subject for his later psychology, I would like to highlight these. The first is listed as 1888b, and the second is included in the clump of articles listed under the heading 1893-94.

[10] It will be included in the new, revised *Standard Edition* that is currently under preparation.

FREUD'S THEORY OF APHASIA REVISITED: EPISTEMOLOGICAL AND CLINICAL IMPLICATIONS

Filip Geerardyn

> Psychoanalysis should be the science of language inhabited by the subject.
> - Jacques Lacan (1981: 243)

Introduction

I would like to open this chapter with a basic question: why study those writings which Freud himself categorised as 'pre-analytical'? What is the purpose of revisiting the pre-analytic Freud? Is it simply for the sake of challenging Freud's authority—a kind of hysterical reaction? After all, he chose not to publish his 'A Project for a Scientific Psychology' (1950), and prevented his monograph *On Aphasia: A Crticial Study* (1953) from being included in his *Collected Writings*.

On the other hand, is the re-visitation of the pre-analytic works merely a means of reducing the origins of psychoanalytic theory, and therefore psychoanalysis itself, to the conceptual frames of which Freud made use—for instance, biology, neurology and neuro-anatomy?[1]

In his book *The Invention of Memory, A New View of the Brain*, Israel Rosenfield states that, whether we realise it ourselves or not, remembering involves the re-organisation of the past:

> A memory only becomes a memory in the context of the present: it is being organised and gets significance within this context. What we remember ourselves, we remember it here and now. (Rosenfield 1988: 81)

Rosenfield shares this point of view with some of the greatest philosophers—Augustine and Nietzsche among them. In this sense, Rosenfield's statement can be seen as a guide to the study of Freud's so-called pre-analytic writings, because his statement also applies to the field of *historiography*. History is always a matter of rewriting the past from a current point of view.

The rehabilitation of aphasia

I shall begin my re-reading of Freud's monograph *On Aphasia* with some preliminary remarks and questions concerning the so-called 'rehabilitation' of aphasia.

It is undeniable that the rehabilitation of aphasia, which is always a laborious and painful process, has specific requirements. Seen from a psychoanalytic point of view, speech therapy, which focuses mainly on impression and 'facilitation' ('*Bahnung*'), bears some striking similarities to the 'talking cure' of psychoanalysis.

It is the characteristically *affective* quality of aphasic speech which attracts special attention. The general psychical state of the aphasic is marked by a fluctuation between what we might call depression and an euphoric state. Frequently, their speech itself is laden with affect. Here we can refer to the well-known aphasic phenomena of swearing, and the powerful 'yes!' and 'no!' which often are the only utterances left in cases of so-called motor aphasia. We can also refer to the nervous, restless quest of the aphasic who attempts to express himself through endless repetition of inadequate circumscriptions. It has been noted, furthermore, that in affective conditions such as anger, the aphasic can suddenly gain access to memories that were thought to be lost.

Such phenomena point towards a relation between affect and speech, as well as between affect and memory. However, it is not at all clear what *kind* of relation. Is the affect a *condition* of remembrance and speech, or are speech and memory actually *disturbed* by the affect?

In addition, the learning process involved in the rehabilitation of aphasia often displays remarkable acceleration, which cannot be explained by facilitation alone.[2] This contradicts the notion of aphasia as a disorder of *memory*, in which it might be asserted that memory images have been destroyed by the brain lesion.

Freud's monograph

These preliminary remarks on the rehabilitation of aphasia evoke Freud's criticism of the theory of *localisation*, as formulated in his monograph *On Aphasia*. In my interpretation of this text I will not deal with the neurological relevance of Freud's critique. This has already been extensively discussed.[3] Instead, I will examine the premises of this form of criticism, or—to put it in other words—Freud's motive or desire.

I wish to demonstrate that his monograph and his critique of the localisation theory were motivated by clinical questions, stemming from his confrontation with hysteria. The problems of speech, language, and the symbolic were attributed a central role in this questioning. I shall argue, therefore, that his monograph is invaluable to the solution of the riddle of Freud's epistemological transition from neurology and neuro-anatomy to psychiatry and psychology, and eventually to psychoanalysis.

One argument for this is easily developed by studying Freud's curriculum. In 1893, in a text written in commemoration of Charcot, Freud indicated that it was his French master who led him in the direction of a psychological explanation of hysteria.[4] One of the methods Charcot frequently used in his clinical demonstrations consisted of the systematic comparison of patients suffering from an organic affection of the nervous system, and hysterical patients—with no evidence of an organic lesion—who at first sight displayed the same clinical picture. The weakest point in Charcot's demonstration was, however, his explanation. Charcot knew perfectly well that his notion of the so-called 'functional' or 'dynamic' lesion was only a rough guess at the cause of the hysterical affections. That cause was searched for in the dynamics of the *'idée-fixe'*, suggestion and autosuggestion—that is, in the *psychological* register of reminiscence and memory. That Charcot himself was aware of the 'inadequacy' of his own explanation is apparent in the way he charged the young Sigmund Freud with the task of finding a conclusive explanation for the difference between the organic and hysterical motor paralyses. After leaving Paris in January 1886, it took Freud seven years to find that explanation. Effectively, Freud 'translated' Charcot's neurophysiological notion of the functional or dynamic lesion into the *psychical* mechanism of repression. Freud published his alternative explanation in 'Some Points for a Comparative Study of Organic and Hysterical Motor Paralyses', in which we find the following words, hinting at this epistemological transition:

> ...and for that purpose I only ask permission to move on to psychological ground—which can scarcely be avoided in dealing with hysteria. (Freud 1893c: 170)

What is this 'psychological ground' to which Freud refers? Most certainly, it is certainly related to *speech*. As Jacques Nassif put it in his seminar on Freud's 'A Project for a Scientific Psychology' (Nassif n.d.), the practice of hypnosis, as employed in Charcot's clinical demonstrations, highlighted the element of speech—or, more accurately, isolated the object of the *voice*. The hysterical symptoms suggested to the subject under hypnosis by Charcot were, then, determined by the spoken words of the master, of 'his master's voice'.

What Freud witnessed during his period of study at the Salpêtrière, then, was not only cases of hysterical conversion, but predominantly cases of what Charcot termed 'hysterical mutism' or 'hysterical aphasia'. Evidence for this can be found in the French edition of Charcot's *Clinical Lectures on the Diseases of the Nervous System* (1887), which Freud was translating into German as early as 1886. This volume contains an appendix with a summary of Charcot's clinical demonstrations on hysterical and organic aphasia during December 1885. Freud implicitly refers to these demonstrations in the letter in which he offers to translate his master's *Lectures*, by saying that as far as his knowledge of the French language is concerned he only suffers from motor aphasia and not from sensory aphasia (Jones 1953: 229).

Charcot explains hysterical aphasia in the same way as hysterical paralyses: 'It is on the cerebral cortex that we must look for the dynamic lesion' (Charcot 1887: 437-8). His interpretation of this 'dynamic lesion' is two-fold. On the one hand, the clinical manifestation of hysterical aphasia seems to be determined by the *idea* which the patients formed for themselves of losing their voice. The exact delineated symptomatology can only be understood as the suggestive effect of the judgement: 'I have no voice', or 'I may not or cannot speak'. Therefore, the hysterical symptom is explained by the *presence of an idea* which is the result of suggestion.

On the other hand, Charcot also comes close to the traditional theory of organic aphasia, which explains speech disorders in terms of a loss in the register of ideas or memory-images. According to this account, hysterics seem to have 'forgotten' how to speak. In hysteria, however, this forgetting is only temporary and therefore cannot be explained by the destruction of brain cells in which the ideas concerned are said to be localised. This explanation can be summed up as follows, then: the hysterical symptom results from the *absence of an idea*.

In the light of this, we should not be too surprised that about halfway between 1886 and 1893 Freud became very interested in the problem of organic aphasia. Ever since the discovery in the brain of Broca's Area (in 1861) and Wernicke's Area (in 1873), speech and its pathology has been explained by this 'presence' or 'absence' of ideas.

By criticising of the theory that specific psychical functions and the functions of speech could be precisely localised in the brain, Freud was proceeding according to the model of his master, Charcot. He contrasted the symptomatology deduced from the schemas of Wernicke and Lichtheim with actual clinical cases he found in medical literature. In this way, Freud supported Eisenlohr's contention that Wernicke and Lichtheim's schema of localised ideas and functions was of 'chiefly didactic value' (Freud 1953: 10).

But for whom is it 'didactic'? The answer is: *for the hysteric.*

By deducing a strict symptomatology from their schema, based on the idea of a strict localisation of specific psychical functions, Wernicke and Lichtheim proceeded in the same way as the hysteric. They produced 'symptoms' which were the result of 'suggestive ideas' they had formed of an affection—that is, aphasia. Their schema does not explain the clinical picture of organic aphasia, but only some forms of hysterical mutism which, like hysterical paralyses, are characterised by 'exact delineation and excessive intensity'. In other words, Wernicke and Lichtheim's localisationalist schema has the same structure as a hysterical symptom—that of the *proton pseudos,* or false connection (*'falsche Verknupfung'*).

Is it too far-fetched to suppose that it was his confrontation with hysteria—with 'excessively intense ideas'—that enabled Freud to recognise the shortcomings of Wernicke and Lichtheim's theory?

This brings me to my second argument concerning Freud's theory of language. After having explored the existent neurological models for the explanation of aphasia, and having criticised them on purely neuro-anatomical grounds, Freud proposed his alternative, *psychological* 'diagram of a word-presentation' (Freud 1915b: 214):

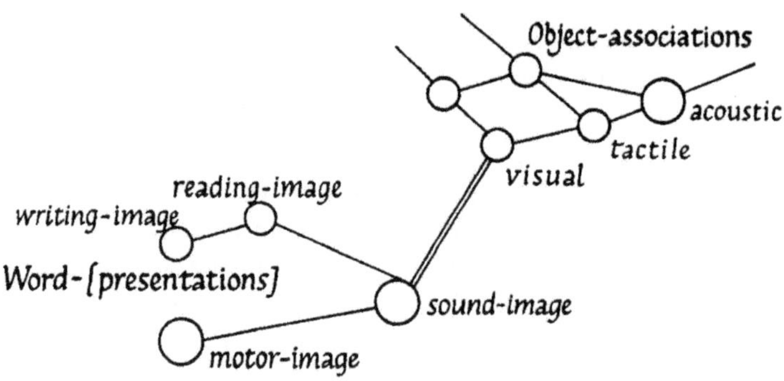

PSYCHOLOGICAL DIAGRAM OF A WORD-PRESENTATION

This consists of two complexes of associated elements which are also linked to each other. His schema represents a speech apparatus which functions as a kind of significance machine: 'The word acquires its significance through its association with the "idea (concept) of the object"' (Freud 1953: 77).

There exists an essential difference between the nature of the 'idea of the object' and that of the 'word-presentation':

> According to philosophical teaching, the idea of the object contains nothing else; the appearance of a 'thing', the 'properties' of which are conveyed to us by our senses, originates only from the fact that in enumerating the sensory impressions perceived from an object, we allow for the possibility of a large series of new impressions being added to the chain of associations (J.S. Mill). This is why the idea of the object does not appear to us as closed, but—indeed—hardly closable, whilst the word-concept appears to us as something that is closed, though capable of extension. (Freud 1953: 78)

This means that Freud's theory of language is threefold. He differentiates between the word-presentation, the object-presentation, and the 'thing'. This 'thing' does not coincide with the idea we retain of the object, as it is always more than what we grasp of it.

What was Freud aiming at with this conception of language and significance? Before answering this question, we must return to Freud's criticism of Wernicke and Lichtheim's speech apparatus. Besides the two 'centre aphasias' (motor and sensory aphasia), Wernicke also postulated the existence of 'conduction aphasia', due to the destruction of the fibre tract between the motor and sensory speech centres. This destruction, according to Wernicke, causes: 'a speech disorder consisting of paraphasia with normal comprehension and articulation, ie., confusion of words and uncertainty in their use' (Freud 1953: 4).

It is this speech disorder which made clear to Freud that Wernicke and Lichtheim's speech apparatus was inadequate and could only be attributed a didactic value. For paraphasia—that is, 'the mistaken use of words'—does not correspond to the possible range of symptoms which can be deduced from it. As Freud indicates, the symptom of paraphasia is also found in cases which cannot be explained by an organic lesion:

> We propose to postpone discussion of the symptom of paraphasia... and also of the reasons which caused Wernicke to regard it as characteristic of an interruption between *a* and *b*. At this stage we only want to mention that the paraphasia observed in aphasic patients does not differ from the incorrect use and the distortion of words which the healthy person can observe in himself in states of fatigue or divided attention or under the influence of disturbing affects,— the kind of thing that frequently happens to our lecturers and causes the listener painful embarrassment. It is tempting to regard paraphasia in the widest sense as a purely functional symptom, a sign of reduced efficiency of the apparatus of speech associations. This does not exclude that they may occur in most typical form as organic focal symptoms. (Freud 1953: 13)

States of fatigue or divided attention, the influence of disturbing affects... these are indeed those circumstances to which we all too readily attribute the cause of our slips of the tongue, and other formations of the unconscious. Here, then, we see Freud focusing upon speech which is disturbed by the affect—*hysterical* speech. In my view, it is this emphasis which forms the motive for his criticism of the localisation theory.

How can this hysterical speech be conceived of, other than as a succession of words, or a substitution of one word for another, between which there yawns a gap, a reference to a 'thing' which always partly escapes symbolisation and can never be totally signified?

In formulating his own theory of hysteria, Freud replaced the medical model by a theory of language. In doing so, he not only deflated the speech apparatus of Wernicke and Lichtheim, but also Charcot's notion of hysteria and Breuer's conception of psychotherapy. For Freud's theory of language took him far beyond the nosographical categories of hysteria formulated by Charcot and Breuer. At this point we can refer to what Freud wrote, a few years later, in the last chapter of the *Studies on Hysteria*, which clearly indicates that he was soon led to make use of Breuer's method in the therapy of *all* neurotic disturbances:

> There is one other advantage in the use of this procedure which I must emphasise. I know of no better way of getting to under-

> stand a severe case of complicated neurosis with a greater or lesser admixture of hysteria than by submitting it to an analysis by Breuer's method. The first thing that happens is the disappearance of whatever exhibits a hysterical mechanism. In the meantime I have learnt in the course of the analysis to interpret the residual phenomena and to trace their aetiology; and in this way I have secured a firm basis for deciding which of the weapons in the therapeutic armory against the neurosis is indicated in the case concerned. When I reflect on the difference that I usually find between my judgement on a case of neurosis before and after an analysis of this kind, I am almost inclined to regard an analysis as essential for the understanding of a neurotic illness. (Breuer & Freud 1895: 266-267)

Conclusion

I have advanced the argument that Freud's point of departure, his '*démarche*', is linguistic, and that it was at the Salpêtrière that he was 'affected' in this direction by the suggestion of Charcot. In the period from 1886 till 1893, during his search for a workable explanation of hysterical symptoms, and through his own confrontation with the clinic of 'excessively intense ideas', Freud succeeded in what we might call his epistemological translation of Charcot's work. This translation consisted of the replacement of neurology by linguistics, a replacement which ironically—but necessarily—undid Charcot's clinical entity of hysteria. For hysteria cannot be explained by the *presence* of an idea, nor by its *absence* (due to the supposed destruction of brain cells), but only by a kind of dialectics *between* presence and absence, as the result of a dynamic process. Freud identified this as the psychical mechanism of repression and of its concomitant—the return of the repressed.

Freud's early subjective linguistics, his 'science of language inhabited by the subject' (Lacan 1981: 243)—in short, the *psychoanalytic theory of language*—may, at least in some aspects, find approval from modern neurology. This has recently been suggested by Rosenfield, in his review of Edelman's theory of neural Darwinism. According to Rosenfield, this theory implies that in order to solve the riddle of memory, we should not focus on the idea of the existence of static reminiscences. We should, instead, concentrate on the dynamic process of *remembering*, which is defined as *the actual reorganising of the past*. Once again, we can refer to a so-called 'pre-analytic' insight of Freud. In the last chapter of *Studies on Hysteria*, he clearly indicates that his 'psychological analysis' or his 'psychotherapy' does not aim for the mere recollection of reminiscences, but for 'the accomplishment of a psychical act which did not take place at the time' (Freud & Breuer 1895: 300).

I believe that a reorganisation of the pre-analytic past of psychoanalysis can provide the impetus for the 'translation' of the so-called 'rehabilitation' of aphasics into a clinic of aphasia. This, just like the clinic of neurosis, is to be conceived of as a clinic of 'excessively intense ideas'. Aphasics realise—at a certain level of rehabilitation—that their lack of words does not simply reflect a loss of memories. Instead, it represents the difficulties they experience with verbalising or symbolising the *affect* released by an organic trauma. For a human being, this can only be represented or mastered on a *psychic* level—that is, through transference. And this is precisely, I believe, the point at which neurology, rehabilitation, and the theory of language and psychoanalysis meet.

Notes

[1] This indeed has been the case on numerous occasions, with varied success. See, for instance, Jones 1953: 415-433; Marcus 1977: xi; Sulloway 1979: 101-131; Hirschmüller 1989: 164; Kris 1954: 25-27; Grünbaum 1984: 3-5; Levin 1978: 152-183.

[2] 'Facilitation' refers here to the process by which, through rehearsal and repetition, the associations between neurons and—hence—between corresponding ideas, is said to be established. In the case of brain damage, a common point of view is that existing facilitations are destroyed. Rehabilitation consists, therefore, in establishing *new* facilitations through rehearsal. However, speech therapists confirm that sudden accelerations in this learning process can only be explained sufficiently by the phenomenon of transference.

[3] For example, in Binswanger 1936, Stengel 1953, and, more recently, Solms & Saling 1990, Rosenfield 1988, and Edelman 1991.

[4] See Freud 1893a.

FREUD'S MERIT AS A PSYCHIATRIST

Hubert Van Hoorde

Introduction

An ancient argument regularly re-surfaces, with an almost discouraging insistence. It serves to remind the analyst—as if a reminder were needed—that misunderstanding or misrecognition (*méconnaissance*) carefully cultivates its points of support.[1]

The argument in question is that Freud was not much of a psychiatrist, and it was due to a lack of intellectual scope that he was impelled to invent psychoanalysis. The critics who support this point of view gloss over the extent of Freud's psychiatric knowledge, alleging that he possessed only a perfunctory understanding of the theories of his time, and that he displayed only a mediocre talent in his practice.

Unfortunately, one cannot contemptuously disregard these arguments, nor simply neutralise them with an opposite assertion. This would merely fall into the trap of opposing a puerile 'oh yes he was a good psychiatrist' to an equally simplistic 'oh no he wasn't, at all!'

The critics

I shall begin by examining two books by Ernst Verbeek, Emeritus Professor of Psychiatry at Ghent University. These works undertake a detailed biographical analysis of Freud, and a reinterpretation of Freud's dreams.

In the first of these works, Verbeek takes up the Oedipus complex. He suggests that Freud, overly anxious to prove the ubiquity of the phenomena with which he was dealing, grossly neglected the profound differences between the clinical categories applicable within psychiatry at the time, and the essential difference between neurotic and normal existence (Verbeek 1971: 7, 12).

This is an idea to which Verbeek returns repeatedly, making various assertions on the theme that 'pathology is totally separate from normality!' (Verbeek 1971: 19). I am not going to dwell upon Verbeek's main concern, which is the nature of Freud's religious beliefs. I shall merely highlight the author's conclusion—that Freud, throughout the course of his life, struggled against *repressed Catholicism*, into which he was initiated (Verbeek alleges) by his nanny, as a child (Verbeek 1971:

52). This state of affairs, according to Verbeek, exposes and explains the roots of the Freudian theory of neurosis, which relies so heavily upon the reunion of the dichotomy between the normal and the pathological.

However, Verbeek regards this theory as resting upon an inadmissible generalisation, because although what Freud says about the psychical apparatus might be applicable to the neurotic that he (Freud) undoubtedly was, it is decidedly *not* applicable to we who are normal, nor to psychotics who are—likewise—qualitatively different. Alongside this argument, Verbeek also airs his views on Freud's personality and the scientificity of his undertakings. He goes so far as to state that Freud failed to avail himself of a scientific methodology, and that he was sadly uncultured (Verbeek 1971: 26).

Verbeek's second book, which deals with Freud's dreams, opens with the interesting assertion that psychiatry has never produced any real geniuses, but if any author could at least lay claim to this status, then it would be Freud (Verbeek 1973: 8). According to Verbeek, the distinctive mark of genius depends on two characteristics. Firstly, the work of a genius must disconcert and remain enigmatic to the reader. Secondly, it must be enduringly original and lively, and never cease to generate novel viewpoints and controversies for successive generations. These two criteria lead Verbeek to a qualified evaluation of Freud's work. Whilst the scales tip in favour of Freud's genius under the second criteria, they tip against him under the first, since—in Verbeek's eyes—Freud's work displays nothing disconcerting or enigmatic (Verbeek 1973: 9). Immediately after this passage, Verbeek resumes his argument concerning Freud's failure to distinguish between the essentially neurotic and non-neurotic.

Indeed, I believe the consistency with which Verbeek strives to uphold the distinction between 'normal' and 'pathological' is significant. Verbeek sketches a portrait of a Freud who—as a neurotic—is socially uncommitted, a half-hearted therapist and unmotivated physician, who despises the whole of humanity and is interested only in people's problems and disorders (Verbeek 1973: 66). There is, thus, a lateral drift evident in Verbeek's criticism of Freud. Whilst, initially, others branded him a pornographer or dirty scribbler, for Verbeek Freud acquires the status of '*salaud*'—in all the senses conveyed by this term.[2] There seems no better word to describe the *dishonesty* Verbeek imputes to Freud. To his mind, Freud was someone who affected secrecy and *did not tell everything* about his dreams, associations, or intimate relationships (Verbeek 1973: 300). Accordingly, Verbeek expresses the opinion that it is only right for us to expect more from a truly great man. It is for this reason that, quoting Binswanger in his foreword, he suggests Freud was a mere amateur in the field of clinical psychiatry.

Verbeek's view exposes the roots of the recurrent opposition in the thinking that underlies negative appraisals of Freud's merit as a psychiatrist. The assumption is that Freud was not conversant with 'major' psychiatry, but dealt only with 'minor' psychiatry—that is, the treatment of the neuroses. However, this does not deter Verbeek from expressing his admiration for Freud's analysis of Schreber. Let us not forget that this reproach is still levelled today at any analyst who chooses *not* to work with psychotics... Unless, of course, he or she is already being criticised for working *with* psychotics—which is also a common complaint!

Unfortunately for several authors, using the Freudian method to ferret out the personality of Freud amounts to an implicit acknowledgement of the validity of that method. This is a point which seems to have been overlooked by quite a number of the opponents of psychoanalysis, although I believe it can be a legitimate critical tactic if carried out appropriately. I want to stress that Verbeek does not fall into this trap: he is fully aware of the psychoanalytic background of his criticism. My main aim here, however, is to trace the origin of the disparagement of Freud's ability as a psychiatrist, and to relate these issues to more general epistemological debates relevant to the practice of psychiatry, irrespective of the historical epoch. In order to work towards this, we must first examine some background details concerning the development of Freud's relationship with psychiatry.

Historical background

Concerning Freud's early medical career, Ernest Jones comments on Freud's 'aversion to the practice of medicine', 'his great liking for his laboratory', and 'his consistent preference for research over mere practice'. Jones was led to conclude that Freud was strongly motivated by a desire 'to discover something new and thus to add to our stock of knowledge' (Jones 1953: 65).

Although Jones is often portrayed as an obsolete hagiographer, the subtlety of his biography never ceases to impress; it is still required reading. It seems to me that his style—which is characterised by an ever-so British sense of understatement, and might be described as 'cool', yet which is nonetheless imbued with admiration for Freud—contributes greatly to the standing of his work. Indeed, one might be tempted to argue for a 'return to Jones' in order to reassess present-day evaluations of Freud.

For instance, Jones writes of Freud that:

> there was the need to discipline himself in scientific method and thus counteract his wilder and more speculative propensities, which dear as they might be could lead him far astray if not controlled. (Jones 1953: 65)

In this very Jonesian paragraph, the record is set straight. Jones observes that Freud cherished his speculative tendencies, but with a sense of deep mistrust. Freud resorted to a scientific method, therefore, as a means of counterbalancing them. Jones's observation also casts light on Freud's desire to excel in his work at the Brücke laboratory. He undertook this pioneering research into the nature of the nervous system in parallel with his studies in medicine. This Jonesian paragraph, then, demonstrates quite graphically what is at stake in the revival of interest in Freud's pre-analytic writings. The early writings illustrate dramatically the struggle between 'speculation' and 'scientific method' which led to the development of psychoanalysis. The importance of these writings for our understanding of the evolution of Freud's thought cannot be overemphasised.

Reluctantly, however, Freud left the Brücke Institute to immerse himself in medical practice. In May 1883, in order to complete his medical studies and acquire the necessary practical experience, he commenced work under Meynert, in Vienna.

Jones paraphrases Freud's view of Meynert from his letters to Martha Bernays:

> Freud agreed with the general opinion that Meynert was the greatest brain anatomist of his time, but he had only a moderate opinion of him as a psychiatrist. (Jones 1953: 72).

Nevertheless, according to Jones, Freud found him a 'stimulating teacher'.[3]

In 1884, Freud returned to the 'Allgemeines Krankenhaus', upon the creation of a department of neurology. He gave lectures as a private tutor ('*Privat-Dozent*') from Spring 1885, and in September of that year his nomination was confirmed by the faculty (Jones 1953: 77).

Neurology, obviously, was still Freud's principal subject at this time. However, let us not forget the fact that the demarcation lines between disciplines were different—or, perhaps, more *permeable*—than they are today. Indeed, even in the present day, few neurologists refrain from enthusiastically practising a psychiatry of their own devising. Nervous diseases are—on the whole—obligingly welcomed into everyday neurological practice. Likewise, it was the lure of the study of nervous diseases—and the influence of Charcot from this field—which set Freud on a new track. His change of course was, in effect, the consequence of a conscious decision. In 1886 Meynert suggested to Freud that he take over the department of neuroanatomy. Freud's visit to Charcot certainly played a major part in his decision to turn down Meynert's offer (Jones 1953: 227).

Although Freud's encounter with Charcot was dominated by ostensibly neuroanatomical concerns, one could argue that it actually redirected Freud towards his passions of yore—the 'speculative tendencies', as Jones described them (Jones 1953: 231).

Borrowing Lacan's notion of logical time, the visit to Charcot could be interpreted as—in effect—'the instant of seeing', *un instant de voir*. Certainly, Charcot enjoyed having all eyes upon him! In the silence of publication which followed Freud took the time for understanding, *le temps de comprendre* (Lacan 1966: 197).[4]

Jones records several very ambitious projects undertaken by Freud in the field of neuroanatomy. Freud began work on several books, hastily writing a few chapters before abandoning them altogether (Jones 1953: 232-233). Clearly, Freud's ambition impelled him to write a general work, in which he would outline his field of study and trace its main ideas. However, it is also apparent that—for Freud—neuroanatomy no longer lent itself to this approach. The reason for this is not that Freud lacked talent, culture or perspicacity. This is soundly contradicted by the quality and importance of his monograph *On Aphasia*.

For the sake of concision, I shall focus only on one aspect of this work: the way in which, for Freud, the notion of *function* itself assumed far greater precedence than the question of *localisation of functions* within the brain. I believe that it is possible to argue that Freud's conception of cerebral function, as set down in the aphasia monograph, differed radically from the ideas of his contemporaries. It provided a *dynamic representation* of mental states which extended far beyond descriptive anatomy.

This tendency is also distinctly in evidence in 'A Project for a Scientific Psychology', where it clearly foreshadows the now familiar ideas Freud would develop on the function of the psyche (Freud 1950: 281-397).

The 'Project', then, in the Lacanian terminology we have adopted, assumes the shape of a *moment de conclure*.[5] Freud has come full circle. His 'psychology for neurologists' can be read as an attempt to attain two goals: firstly, to arrive at an understanding of the *modus operandi* of the psyche; secondly, an attempt to solve the insoluble, to envisage the means by which psychical functions are articulated around cerebral or neurocellular mechanisms. The fact that the *Project* was never published, however, reveals that Freud was not at all satisfied with his efforts, and that he believed he had not brought his ideas to their appropriate conclusion.[6]

So what was Freud's relationship with the psychiatry of his time? In 1886 he established himself as a specialist in nervous diseases (*'Nervenartz'*) in Vienna. From what he wrote of this period in his 1925b *An Autobiographical Study*, his preoccupations were initially of a therapeutic order. This would seem often the case with anyone who at some stage in their career ventures into the study of psychiatry. Freud wrote:

> My therapeutic arsenal contained only two weapons, electrotherapy and hypnotism, for prescribing a visit to a hydropathic establishment after a single consultation was an inadequate source of income. (Freud 1925b: 16)

However, Freud soon came to realise the inefficiency of electrotherapy, and the danger of hypnotism. 'For the first time there was a sense of having overcome one's helplessness'—he comments ironically—'and it was highly flattering to enjoy the reputation of being a miracle-worker' (Freud 1925b: 17).

At this time there was a gap in medicine, which needed to be filled on both a therapeutic and a theoretical plane: Freud himself uses the word *'Lücke'* or 'gap'. At first he believed it was filled by the discovery of the sexual roots of neurosis. He states in the same article that filling the gap in medicine quieted his medical conscience. In that gap would lie the very essence of the Freudian approach, as we will argue further on.

Psychiatry in this period was characterised by a desire to found itself upon the natural sciences. Roughly speaking, this had resulted in two approaches: the localisation of psychical functions, and the elaboration of a taxonomic system of disorders.[7] At its outset, this young science had striven to attain status within the field of medicine, as opposed to philosophy and psychology.[8] The social and scientific status of psychiatry was, therefore, very far removed from what some historical events—which are now regarded with a form of poetic exaggeration—appear to suggest. For instance, events such as Pinel's refusal to shackle the insane, and Joseph Guislain's architectural humanisation of the notion of the asylum.[9]

The state of psychiatry in this stage of Freud's career was by no means propitious, and we might be inclined to accept that Freud was fully aware of this. As Hirschmüller has observed, the psychiatric curriculum with which Freud was confronted during his stay with Meynert did not exactly stimulate his interest. Rather, it prompted him to turn his attention away from psychiatry and to follow an entirely new course (Hirschmüller 1991: 108-210). Indeed, Hirschmüller's evaluation of Meynert is suggestive. The institute in which Meynert was active was an organicist psychiatric school which enjoyed an international reputation. But although it was dedicated to the development of medicine based on the natural sciences, Meynert's system of thought was—according to Hirschmüller—'more dogmatic than empirically oriented' (Hirschmüller 1991: 223-224). Freud's visit to Paris would bring him into contact with a dynamic conception of psychical disorders, in which the methods of pathological anatomy would prove of no use whatsoever.

Theoretical elaboration

We are confronted with the fact that psychiatry developed against the background of the nascent medical clinic. Emancipating itself from previous theoretical speculations, medicine was revamped by the clinic as a science of the particular which provides access to the general.[10]

Clinical science, however, possesses a distinctive feature. It is founded upon the *sign* and the *gaze*; it concerns the *scopic* field. In psychiatry, this led to an increasing concern with anatomical features. The subject of psychiatry was left behind as a kind of residue, for the subject always eludes the objectification of medical discourse, carrying his ailments with him. Traditionally, the subject's symptoms were collected by the psychiatrist in the form of *case histories*.[11] The examination of cases, the meticulous recording of the life-story of a subject, can be seen in the work of Pinel, Kretschmer[12] or—indeed—even in Jacques Lacan's psychiatric work.[13]

By its nature, the case-historical approach always results in a 'successful' conclusion. However, sometimes it may cave in under the weight of its own casuistry, and expose the underlying impression of a mere recording of disparate elements. In my view, there are two possible outcomes to this *aporia*. One can either opt to construct an increasingly refined and complicated taxonomy (this was the path chosen by psychiatrists such as Kraepelin and Kretschmer), or one can veer towards the clinic of the *signifier*.

This was the conclusion Lacan reached in his psychiatric thesis of 1932, thereby following in the footsteps of Freud. As Panhuysen shows, it is apparent that Freud was—initially—looking for an answer to the psychiatric *aporia* of his time by concentrating his efforts on taxonomies and systems (Panhuysen 1990: 91). Having first abandoned large-scale projects in the field of anatomy, Freud proceeded with his study of hysteria—the results and development of which are now familiar. Nevertheless, he continued to contemplate writing a *general theory* of the neuroses. Freud's correspondence with Fliess is an adumbrated project of this kind.[14] But—once again—this was an undertaking which was not followed to a conclusion, and never progressed beyond the stage of a 'project'. This strongly suggests, then, that Freud realised the taxonomic route was a dead-end.

At this point a paradox emerges. Had Freud been the accomplished psychiatrist which some critics have reproached him for not being, then he might simply have behaved as a theoretician of his time. He would have chosen the taxonomic route and produced conventional work on the neuroses which would—doubtlessly—be forgotten today, as are the works by even his most outstanding colleagues. If he had opted for the orthodox, he would have bypassed psychoanalysis.

However, this paradox stems from the fact that Freud distanced himself from the traditional praxis and theory of his time. Rather than losing the subject as a 'residue', Freud's stance enabled him to rescue the subject. Freud gathered together the remnants that the so-called science of psychiatry had produced by objectifying the patient, reducing the patient to a tabulated element in its over-arching taxonomy. Panhuysen vividly exposes the difference between Kraeplin—a builder of systems—and Freud, who devoted his attention to *psychical causality* (Panhuysen 1990: 126).

In contemporary terms, to state that Freud dealt with 'psychical causality' is—in effect—to state that he immersed himself in the clinic of the signifier, an approach which recognises the import of *transference*. This was Freud's own creation, the fruit of an epistemological imperative. The clinic of the *sign* (as opposed to the clinic of the *signifier*), supported by a semiological approach, produced a residue with which it was unable to cope: the subject and his (life-) story. This residue, however, was the very substance of the ensuing clinic inaugurated by Freud, as a substitute for the *aporia* of traditional psychiatry.

Needless to say, these issues are still far from being resolved. As I write, the landslide is still taking place. The way in which psychiatry is still cramped within the neo-Kraepelian taxonomy, characterised by an increasingly invasive DSM system, raises the question whether it can legitimately claim status—or even the right to exist. I would argue that psychiatry itself exists merely by virtue of the lack around which it is structured—which in turn emerges as a consequence of the stubbornness of the methods it employs.

Psychoanalysis is a response to this lack. However, it does not fill it, since it deals with the subject as a divided subject. Freud's placement of the divided subject at the centre of his new science, independent of psychiatry, was—let us not forget—the cause of much scandal, as was its focus on sexuality.

Conclusion

I shall now summarise the epistemological processes which demarcate the sphere of psychiatry. As a clinical science, psychiatry is characterised within the field of medicine by its object—the subject and his language. This object is thus of a *historical* order, and cannot be reduced to the rank of an object of observation or experimentation—as is the case in the natural sciences. Even if such observations or experiments were possible, an irreducible residue subsists which—due to the action of the unconscious—*divides* both the patient and the physician. Hence, a clinical psychiatry cannot be conceived of as operating outside the bounds of the transference phenomenon.

The point of departure for *any form of psychiatry as a clinical practice* is the case-study. In this respect, psychiatry has developed upon the foundations of the medical clinic, which was a product of the previous century. This clinic can be described as a clinic of the gaze or—in other terms—a clinic of the *sign*. This is in opposition to the clinic of the *signifier*, which is elaborated in Lacan's psychoanalytic theorisations.

Three positions can be distinguished. Firstly, 'the clinic *with* the signifier'. This is a clinic which avails itself of signifiers—such as the diagnosis—which it appends to the patient. This position breaks apart, however, and leads to the second—'the clinic of the *sign*'. Here, concern is upon a search for the signs of the disease, and for a semiology which lends itself to a systemic approach. However, in psychiatry, there also exists a branch of the clinic of the sign which uses the signifier without theorising it. This results in a clinic of the history of subjective suffering. This clinic inevitably veers towards the third position—'the clinic of the *signifier*'. Here, the patient's signifiers constitute the material from which the main signifier which holds sway over the neurosis might be grasped. It is this position which serves the function of a science of the subject.

Any return to 'the clinic with the signifier' is a regression, by means of which the psychiatrist avoids coming face to face with the history and suffering emanating from the subject. This is also true of the simple application of signifiers borrowed from a science, but which are devoid of any reference to the patient's own signifiers. An approach of this kind functions as a damper; it operates in the manner of those causalistic myths which cloak the divided nature of the subject.

The psychical apparatus is not conceivable without a biological or somatic substratum. Anatomical and physiological disorders of this substratum find expression as psychical disorders at the level of the psyche. However, this logic does not apply to all psychical disorders. In the case of the subject and his suffering, it is the signifier which performs the role of substratum. To approach the problem of the structure of this state of affairs entails taking into account the unconscious, and the insertion of the subject into language or the symbolic order. In this context, the importance of the subject and his 'life-story' cannot be overemphasised.

These principles—from the perspective of psychiatry—would entail a partitioning of the clinical field. A clinic of the sign—resting on a somato-physiological substratum—would co-exist alongside a clinic of the signifier, the substratum of which is psychical—that is, encompassed by the signifier. In order to negotiate these two fields appropriately, it should be remembered that the first finds expression through the second. Thus, it is advisable to make the subject and his life-history the object of psychiatry. Furthermore, human suffering is inextricably linked to the human condition—that is, to the discomfort attendant upon the advent of the subject. The asymmetry of these two clinical fields betokens the lack which occupies a central position in psychiatry. As a clinical science, psychiatry is founded upon this lack, and echoes the fact that the subject is only a subject on account of the division he suffers.

The two criticisms of Freud with which I began this investigation—that Freud was neurotic and a mediocre psychiatrist—stem from a dual misapprehension. Firstly, promulgation of a dichotomy between the 'normal' and the 'pathological' arises from the *'méconnaissance'* of the divided subject.[15] Secondly, the fundamental disharmony inherent in the psychiatric field has been glossed over.

The accusation of lack of imagination levelled at Freud is exposed as a ploy to conceal a more pertinent lack in psychiatry itself, which Freud tackled by moving away from the position of interrogator, in order to adopt the role of listener. In effect, Freud is imputed to have gone outside the bounds of psychiatry whereas, in actuality, psychiatry *prevented* him from practising his profession.

Notes

1 See Evans 1996. He states in his *An Introductory Dictionary of Lacanian Psychoanalysis* under the heading *'méconnaissance'*, that this French term corresponds roughly to the English words 'misunderstanding' and 'misrecognition', but 'is usually left untranslated when translating Lacan into English in order to show its close relationship with the term *connaissance* (knowledge)' (Evans 1996: 109).

2 The term *'salaud'* is used here with the connotations given to it by the French philosopher Jean-Paul Sartre. The particular relation a *'salaud'* has with his truth, and with truth in general, as well as his lack of commitment to his fellow man, are all implied here.

3 A thorough examination of this episode can be found in Hirschmüller 1989.

4 See Evans 1996 for more detail, from whose *Dictionary* I take this quotation: 'In the 1945 paper, Lacan argues that logical time has a tripartite structure, the three moments of which are: (i) the instant of seeing; (ii) the time for understanding; (iii) the moment of concluding. By means of a sophism (the problem of the three prisoners) Lacan shows how these three moments are constructed not in terms of objective chronometric units but in terms of an intersubjective logic based on a tension between waiting and haste, between hesitation and urgency. Logical time is thus "the intersubjective time that structures human action" (Lacan 1966: 75)' (Evans 1996: 206).

5 See footnote 4.

6 It should be noted here that the publication of the *Project* at a later date was the cause of some controversy in the world of psychiatry. The *Project* had barely been translated when it was harshly reviewed with somewhat ill-placed and even insidious arguments. This pro-

voked me into what was (I readily concede) a rather polemical reaction. See Jongerius 1992, and Van Hoorde 1993. Criticism of the *Project* rested upon a rather odd argument—that as Freud himself had not (over the course of forty years) decided to publish this work, then it was not necessary to take the trouble of translating and publishing it for modern readers. It was also argued that the work brought nothing new to light, and was not particularly interesting. Such an evaluation is now hard to believe. What is even more incredible, most commentators seemed oblivious to the fact that the work articulates a major epistemological shift.

7 See Van de Vijver & Geerardyn 1992b: ix.

8 See Sauret 1993.

9 Philippe Pinel (1745-1826) was the first French psychiatrist to present a coherent theory of insanity in his *Traité médico-philosophique sur l'aliénation mentale ou la manie*, published in Paris in the year IX, ie. 1802. He initiated the 'traitement moral' in France and had a strong belief in the medical approach along humanistic lines of the treatment of insanity. Joseph Guislain (1797-1860) was born in Ghent and was the Belgian counterpart of Pinel. He described himself as 'a physician by profession and architect by choice'. He was the first professor to teach psychiatry at the University of Ghent. He proposed a theory of insanity as well as plans for a model asylum—which earned him a royal prize—in his major work, the *Leçons orales sur les phrénopathies, ou traité théorique et pratique des maladies mentales*. For more information about Guislain, see Evrard 1995.

10 The nascent medical clinic opened a radical new field, by permitting *a scientific discourse on the individual*—ignoring Aristotle's decree to the contrary: 'L'*objet* du discours peut aussi bien être un *sujet*, sans que les figures de l'objectivité soient pour autant altérées. C'est cette réorganisation *formelle* et *en profondeur*, plus que l'abandon des théories et des vieux systèmes, qui a ouvert la possibilité d'une *expérience clinique*; elle a levé le vieil interdit aristotélicien: on pourra enfin tenir sur l'individu un discours à structure scientifique' (Foucault 1988: x).

11 See Van Hoorde 1992.

12 Ernst Kretschmer (1888-1964) was a German psychiatrist (Marburg and Tübingen) who wrote meticulous case studies and developed on that basis a new syndrome (*'der sensitive Beziehungswahn'*) which attacked Kraepelin's nosology. He is also known for his typology.

13 See Lacan 1975.

14 See, for instance, Masson 1985: 69-71.

15 See footnote 1, above.

THE PLACE OF COCAINE IN THE WORK OF FREUD

Rik Loose

> This is the malady in them all for which law must find a pharmacon. Now it is a sound old adage that it is hard to fight against two enemies at once—even when they are enemies from opposite quarters. We see the truth of this in medicine and elsewhere. (Plato, Laws, 919b)

> There is no such a thing as a harmless remedy. The *pharmakon* can never be simply beneficial. (Derrida 1972: 69-198)

Introduction

In *An Autobiographical Study* Freud describes his involvement with the drug cocaine as a 'side interest, though it was a deep one...' (Freud 1925b: 14). In the short passage he dedicates to this period of his life, he refers only to the missed opportunity of discovering cocaine as a local anaesthetic. Freud seems to marginalise this aspect of his work, as—indeed—have many others. When it is not marginalised by others, it is often used as a way of denigrating his work. It has been argued, for instance, that Freud was addicted to cocaine, and that the founding texts of psychoanalysis were a result of grandiose delusions induced by the drug.[1] On occasion, serious studies of this period in Freud's work have been undertaken.[2] These studies insist on the importance of a return to, and a thorough exploration of, this aspect of Freud's work. Their aim is to reassess the problematic relationship which has existed between psychoanalysis and addiction from its very beginning. A return to the cocaine episode would be fruitful if we acquired something new from it—if not new answers then, at least, some new questions regarding the way in which the problem of the addictions can be situated within psychoanalysis.

In this paper, I shall read Freud's *Cocaine Papers* as a beginning of the Freudian adventure. An exploration of certain aspects of his subsequent trajectory—until the so-called 'birth' of psychoanalysis in 1900, with the *Interpretation of Dreams*—will allow us to establish a relationship between these papers by Freud and concepts such as 'the sexual toxins', 'libido' and 'the actual neuroses'.

A 'side interest'?

Freud's *Cocaine Papers* make interesting reading in themselves, but especially within the context of his other work—that is, not as a 'side interest' of Freud, nor as an 'allotrion', which is the term he used to classify his interest in cocaine in a letter to Wittels. 'Allotrion' is an interesting word. It can be defined as a rupture, the introduction of a foreign idea into the body of ideas within a certain scientific discourse or doctrine. F. Geberovich makes the interesting observation that a closely associated French term—*'allotriophagie'*—signified, during Freud's time: 'The deprivation of appetite due to the incorporation of non-alimentary substances' (Geberovich 1984: 158-159). Freud's choice of words may not have been accidental, but was perhaps motivated unconsciously. Jones refers to Freud's conspicuous 'irrationalities'—such as forgetting, mistakes and lapses—on the rare occasions he wrote about this episode in his life (Byck 1974: 200). We know that it is precisely these which reveal an unconscious desire unsuccessfully censored. In other words, it is possible that Freud repressed something concerning this episode in his life.

In seminar XI, Jacques Lacan suggests: 'The truth is perhaps simply one thing, namely the desire of Freud himself, the fact that something in Freud was never analysed' (Lacan 1979: 12). He continues:

> What I had to say on the Names-of-the-Father had no other purpose, in fact, than to put into question the origin, to discover by what privilege Freud's desire was able to find the entrance into the field of experience he designates as the unconscious. It is absolutely essential that we should go back to this origin if we wish to put analysis on its feet. (Lacan 1979: 12)

On the next page, Lacan asserts that this question of Freud's desire is not to be considered on a psychological level, that is, as a trait of his individual personality. Freud's desire concerns desire in the position of an object, and as caused by an object. This object is the unconscious and so, therefore, *Freud's unconscious*. Freud's life and his work cannot be considered as separate entities. One of the first objects of Freud's interest was the drug cocaine. In fact, we know from certain letters he wrote to his fiancée Martha, and from reading 'Über Coca' (the first of these papers), that he was very passionate about cocaine (Byck 1974:

39-45; 48-73). It seems to me, then, that Freud's relationship to the drug is an area of research which opens the door to an understanding of his discovery of the unconscious, and the nature of the object in psychoanalysis. Perhaps it also sheds some light upon the virtual exclusion of the problem of addiction from this field of research.

Two observations

At this point I want to introduce two observations which seem paradoxical:

- Despite Freud's personal and professional encounter with drugs and addiction, this clinical problem has remained a relatively unexplored aspect of his work.

- In his postscript to *The Question of Lay Analysis,* Freud writes that he was never a doctor in the proper sense of 'medical activity', and that he was never aware of any craving to help suffering humanity, because his innate sadistic disposition was not strong enough. When prompted by fresh influences, he became interested in the neuroses, though he felt that his lack of medical temperament was no obstacle to the treatment of his patients—rather, the contrary (Freud 1926: 253-254).

However, in a letter of 25th May 1884, to Martha Bernays, Freud refers to the role cocaine played in the discovery of his medical vocation. He wrote: 'It is only now I feel like a doctor, because I have been able to help a patient and I hope to help others' (Byck 1974: 7). In other words, Freud wanted to cure patients of their suffering *medically,* and he hoped he had found a panacea in cocaine which would enable him to achieve this.

The difference between this and his later position is that, later, his desire was to cure *analytically,* via psychological methods, without dependency upon a pharmaceutical object. Earlier, he had placed all his hopes on the drug cocaine.

Freud suggested that a conscious wish to help could be the transformation of an unconscious sadistic impulse or desire. It was, perhaps, this same unconscious impulse which played a role in his relationship with his friend and colleague, Ernst von Fleischl-Marxow. At the same time, Fleischl played the role of Freud's rival and ego-ideal.

He died of a cocaine overdose, after Freud had prescribed the drug in order to wean him from a morphine addiction.

The real difference between Freud's earlier and later positions is that, in the interim period, he had discovered unconscious desire. He had also discovered that the object which causes this desire is—by its nature—a *lost object*. This lost object forms the object of psychoanalysis, in stark contrast to Freud's initial wish that cocaine—as an object—would serve the function of an ideal therapeutic instrument.

Vera Ocampo summarises the consequences of Freud's encounter with cocaine as follows:

> The encounter with the drug awakes in Freud the desire to cure others and himself [his neurasthenic and neurotic symptoms], which from the beginning emerge as two sides of the same medal; the first other of this Freudian desire is an addict Fleischl; the problematic nature of addiction leads to a therapeutic act in which for the first time Freud questions his own desire and further at the heart of his intellectual adventure, the question of desire itself; but if addiction is the first object of Freud's desire to cure it also constitutes his first obstacle and his first therapeutic failure. (Ocampo 1989: 115-116)

So what was the consequence of Freud's failure with cocaine? To answer this question it is necessary to re-trace some of Freud's epistemological steps. It is hoped that this chapter might form the beginning of a research project concerning the question of how the addictions—theoretically and clinically—should be situated within the Freudian field.

By choosing to explore Freud's work—rather than his personal life—we avoid the risk of reducing the *Cocaine Papers* to a mere moment in Freud's biography. As with all Freud's scientific achievements, there is more involved than his personal history. Jean Allouch—for instance—seems to suggest that if we consider Freud's relationship to the drug cocaine as a symptom, then the necessity of this symptom will be reflected in his writings about it (Allouch, 1984: 28). We know that Freud's symptom 'ceased to write itself'; he dropped his passionate relationship with cocaine and this opened up other pathways. A detailed study of Freud's writings on cocaine is therefore vital to an understanding of these pathways.

The Cocaine Papers

The text 'Über Coca' which came first in the series, published in July 1884, is a curious mixture of objective scientific writing and a subjective writing, and reflects a passionate belief in the magical properties of the drug. Freud begins with a botanical description, followed by a historical overview of its use in Peru and its reception in Europe. He continues with a look at the effects of cocaine on animals and the human body, before concluding with an exploration of several therapeutic possibilities. The properties of cocaine which initially attracted Freud to the drug were its ability to increase the capacity for work, to allow people to do without food for longer periods, and to increase physical strength. In response to Poeppig's description of physical and intellectual decadence as a result of habitual cocaine use, Freud wrote that 'all other observers affirmed that the use of coca in moderation is more likely to promote health than to impair it, and that the coqueros live to a great age' (Byck 1974: 52).

When Freud refers to experiments with cocaine on himself and others, he mentions that individuals react differently to the drug. He acknowledges that there is no uniform effect. Freud returns to this in his subsequent papers on the drug. In the last paper—'Craving for and fear of Cocaine'—he relates the variable effects of cocaine to individual variations in excitability and 'a factor of individual predisposition' (Byck 1974: 175). It was this lack of uniform effect which shattered Freud's medical-pharmacological fantasy of finding a universal panacea for human suffering.

Pharmacology relies on two related factors. Firstly, the predictability of the effects of drugs and, secondly, the lack of difference in reaction to them between individuals and within individuals. Freud's emphasis on the *instability* of the effect of cocaine contradicts the suggestion by the editor of the *Cocaine Papers*, Robert Byck, that Freud was interested in the science of pharmacology and could be considered one of its founders (Byck 1974: xvii). This is not to say that Freud was not interested in cocaine as a therapeutic instrument. He considered in some depth the various therapeutic possibilities of cocaine, and his interest in the use of cocaine endured for some time. However, his very first scientific observations had already begun to subvert his personal and medical fantasy of cocaine as the ideal pharmacological instrument. Indeed, it was this 'working-through' of the fantasy which resulted in the abandonment of cocaine as an object.

Writing on the *psychical* effects of cocaine in 'Über Coca', Freud mentions that the exhilaration and lasting euphoria do not appear to differ from the normal euphoria of a healthy person. The mood induced by cocaine gives Freud the impression that the drug does not stimulate in a direct way, but affects those elements in our general state of well-being which lead to depression. He writes, somewhat enigmatically:

> One may perhaps assume that the euphoria resulting from good health is also nothing more than the normal condition of a well-nourished cerebral cortex which is 'not conscious of the organs of the body to which it belongs. (Byck 1974: 60).

In this euphoric state, produced by the effect of cocaine, long-lasting, intensive mental and physical work can be performed without fatigue, and without the need for much food and sleep. Freud wonders why and how cocaine can have this stimulating effect. Through various authors, he considers the possible relationships between cocaine and three interrelated elements, in order to determine *where* the effect of cocaine takes place. These elements are:

- the system or organism into which the cocaine can be incorporated;
- a vital energy contained within this organism, which can be affected by this incorporation, and;
- the conversion of this energy into work.

Where does cocaine intervene? *How* does it intervene? These questions emerge within the theoretical framework of nineteenth century energetics, which is based on the principle (or law) that the total amount of energy in an isolated system (or organism) is constant. Freud attempts to answer these questions within that framework. One consideration is that cocaine can be a 'source of savings'. He writes:

> A system which has absorbed even an extremely small amount of cocaine is capable, as a result of the reaction of the body to coca, of amassing a greater store of vital energy which can be converted into work than would have been possible without coca. If we take the amount of work as being constant, the body which has absorbed cocaine should be able to manage with a

> lower metabolism, which in turn means a smaller intake of food. (Byck 1974: 68)

Cocaine, then, accumulates disposable energy in the organism. Therefore, if this energy is not being used the organism will need less food and sleep. Freud writes that this does not necessarily contradict the law of conservation of energy. He explains this as follows

> For labour which draws upon food or tissue components involves a certain loss, either in the utilisation of assimilated food or in the conversion of energy into work; this loss could perhaps be reduced if certain appropriate steps were taken. (Byck 1974: 68)

Freud does not explain what these steps are and how they work. Here it seems as if he is forcing himself to stay within the limited theoretical framework of nineteenth century energetics.

As a next step, Freud considers the possibility that the influence of cocaine results in providing a better availability of materials already stored in the organism, which thus produces more working power and necessitates less food. Freud considers this next step because experiments on animals have refuted the conception of cocaine as a 'source of savings'. Animals which had been given cocaine succumbed quicker to inanimation (or energy loss) than those who had received no cocaine. However, Freud suggests that an accidental experiment of history contradicts this conclusion. In the year 1781 the city of La Paz was under siege. Only those inhabitants who had taken cocaine survived starvation. Could there be a difference between animals and human beings in terms of their reaction to cocaine? And if so, what is that difference?

Freud is unable to answer these questions. This prompts him to conclude merely that: 'The therapeutic quality of coca which we took as our argument at the onset does not, therefore, deserve to be rejected out of hand' (Byck 1974: 69).

Evidently, Freud is not yet prepared to give up his fantasy of cocaine as panacea, even though he has been unable to answer several crucial questions within the conceptual framework of his time. However, on the question of the survival of the starving cocaine-users of La Paz, Freud comments:

> In this connection one might recall the fact that the human nervous system has an undoubted if somewhat obscure, influence on the nourishment of tissues; psychological factors, after all, cause a healthy man to lose weight. (Byck 1974: 69)

Are these 'psychological factors' a first indication of a way out of the theoretical framework of energetics? In fact, Freud has still some way to go before he is able to arrive at this point.

In the 'Addenda' to 'Über Coca', Freud writes that the only constant effect of cocaine he had found was an increased capacity for work (Byck 1974: 107). This led him to the idea of a series of experiments to demonstrate the effect of cocaine through comparing the variations of certain measurable quantities in living beings. In his paper 'Contribution to the Knowledge of the Effect of Cocaine', Freud wrote that he expected a greater uniformity in the action of cocaine where an objective method of measurement was used (Byck 1974: 98). Freud wanted to investigate the motor power of certain muscle groups and psychic reaction time as operationalisations of the action of cocaine. For this, he used respectively a dynamometer and a neuro-amoebimeter. He carried out these experiments on himself, because he said he had such a regular reaction to cocaine, unlike most other people. Freud continued to experiment over a period of weeks. It is important to follow these experiments step by step, rather than concentrating only upon the general conclusions which Freud drew from them.

The first experiments showed that cocaine caused a marked increase in motor power. He also noticed something else, namely, that there were daily fluctuations and fluctuations between days, in terms of motor power. In other words, there was another variable at work.

This radically changed the situation. To Freud it now appeared impossible to measure the effect of cocaine independently from the interference of this (as yet) unknown factor. Nevertheless, Freud continued his measurements of motor energy. This time, however, *without* the influence of cocaine. He was struck by two facts:

> Firstly, the figures for the motor energy of a muscle group reveal a regular fluctuation in the course of a day; secondly, the same figures reach quite different absolute values on different days. (Byck 1974: 101)

These findings, then, led Freud to conclude that the variations in motor energy are an expression of a 'general state of well-being', and not an effect of cocaine. The magical properties of cocaine are beginning to break down. Freud continued by suggesting that he did not consider the action of cocaine to be direct, but *indirect*, and affected by an improvement of the state of well-being (Byck 1974: 102). This is supported, according to Freud, by two factors:

> Muscular energy increases most obviously after taking cocaine when cocaine euphoria has developed, but before the total quantity can be absorbed into the circulation; and motor power increases considerably if the cocaine takes effect when the general condition is poor and motor power diminished. (Byck 1974: 102)

Freud proved experimentally what he had briefly suggested in 'Über Coca', namely, that the mood induced by cocaine is not so much due to direct stimulation as to the *disappearance* of those factors in our 'general state of well-being' which cause depression (Byck 1974: 60). Cocaine has an optimum effect when the condition is poor (depression), and its effect is less when the condition is normal (a good mood). The effect comes about via a state of euphoria and not as a result of the direct effect of the substance on the organism. Cocaine affects those factors which make the difference between a good mood and a bad mood.

So, to his three elements (organism, vital energy, and work) Freud added a fourth: a factor (or factors) which causes variations in a 'general state of well-being'. Cocaine, when incorporated by the organism, results in more muscular energy (and work capacity) due to a factor which can cause variations in a 'general state of well-being'.

Allouch writes that cocaine does not act upon a constant, but on something which is variable (Allouch 1984: 41). Towards the end of the paper on his experiments, Freud draws similar conclusions from his investigation of the influence of cocaine upon reaction time. These later experiments confirm his earlier findings. What follows proves very important. He writes:

> I often noticed that under cocaine my reaction times were shorter and more uniform than before taking the drug; but sometimes, in a more cheerful and efficient mood, my psychic reactions were just as good. (Byck 1974: 104)

In other words, certain psychical conditions such as 'feeling well' or a 'good mood', have the same effect as cocaine. A condition of well-being, such as a good mood or euphoria, resulted in similar quantities of disposable motor energy to the effect of cocaine.

On the basis of his results, it would seem likely that cocaine would have become less important to Freud as an object of scientific interest and research. He had discovered that it was nothing more than a remedy for a 'weak psychic state'. As such, it had lost its privileged place as the only relevant factor in the phenomena he was investigating. The 'psychic state' and its 'weakness' turned out to be the most relevant variables. Later they became the prime objects of his interest and research.

However, the status of cocaine as a fantasy object for Freud had not yet ceased to write itself in his work, even though the subversion of the fantasy continued in the scientific advances he continued to make.

In March 1885, about three months after the paper on his experiments, Freud read a paper before the Psychiatric Society of Vienna. In this paper, he summarised his findings. Before discussing cocaine as a means of weaning morphine addicts from their drug, he mentions another use which is of direct interest to psychiatry:

> Psychiatry is rich in drugs that can subdue over-stimulated nervous activity, but deficient in agents that can heighten the performance of the depressed nervous system. It is natural therefore, that we should think of making use of the effects of cocaine that we have described above in the forms of illness, that we interpret as states of weakness and depression of the nervous system without organic lesions. As a matter of fact, cocaine has been used since its discovery against hysteria, hypochondria, etc. (Byck 1974: 116)

Here we can see that Freud wanted to hold on to the belief that cocaine was therapeutically useful. But, this time, as a psychopharmacological remedy for a state of 'psychic weakness', which is *not* caused by organic lesions. The drug works because its general effect in cases of psychic weakness is euphoria. However, Freud is left with the question of why it proves effective in cases of psychic illness, of which hysteria is one instance. Jean Allouch writes that—at this point in Freud's work—there, where cocaine was, shall psychoanalytic treatment come to be (Allouch 1984: 40). That is to say, for Freud cocaine also functioned as a therapeutic solution to the problem of hysteria (amongst other problems), as well as a means by which he began to question the nature of hysteria. It is interesting to note that it was in his work on cocaine that the functions of therapy and scientific research (or theory) first came together, an ethical position he would maintain for the rest of his life.

Alongside this, Freud's reference to 'states of weakness and depression without organic lesions' seems to indicate a major shift in his thinking. In the years 1882 to 1885, Freud received a thorough training in neuroanatomical and neurophysiological thinking from teachers such as Nothnagel, Meynert and Brücke. Within this theoretical framework, hysteria and other forms of 'psychic weakness' were caused by an organic lesion. This concept of 'organic lesion' served to explain totally—and to unify—the whole field of afflictions of the nervous system. In 1885, when speaking to the Psychiatric Society of Vienna about the general effect of cocaine, Freud began to refer to afflictions of the nervous system which were *not* based on organic lesions. The implication is that he was now entertaining the idea of psychic processes as the basis for nervous illnesses. He had broken through the framework of organic-physiological thinking, with its implicit reliance on the principle of conservation of energy as formulated by Helmholtz. We have seen how this fundamental principle functioned as a conceptual 'straightjacket', when Freud tried to understand and explain, scientifically, the effects of cocaine on the human body and the results of his experiments on cocaine.

Freud's passionate interest in cocaine, and his ongoing scientific work, led him to the discovery of psychic processes and a desire to understand their different ways of functioning. This was without the loss of his commitment to therapy, which he sustained throughout his encounter with the drug.

We shall take one final step with Freud in order to account for his complete abandonment of cocaine as a therapeutic object and as his object of medical fantasy. In July 1887 he wrote his final paper on the subject, entitled, 'Craving for and Fear of Cocaine'. In the interim he had become interested in hysteria and had visited Charcot in Paris. The German psychiatrist Erlenmeyer had accused Freud of contributing to the proliferation of cocaine addiction (Byck 1974: 172). Erlenmeyer described cocaine addiction as 'the third scourge of mankind', alongside alcohol and morphine addiction. Robert Byck encourages us to read this final paper as Freud's reply to the accusation. However, the danger of this reading is that it tends to overlook the significance of the epistemological shift in Freud's view of the drug. It was this which shattered his medical fantasy for once and for all.

In this final paper, Freud argues that the value of cocaine for morphine addicts is negligible, because it would simply become a *substitute* for morphine. In response to the mass hysteria concerning the dangers of cocaine, he writes:

> All reports of addiction to cocaine and deterioration resulting from it refer to morphine addicts, persons who already in the grip of one demon are so weak in will power, so susceptible, that they would misuse, and indeed have misused, any stimulant held out to them. Cocaine has claimed no other, no victim on its own. (Byck 1974: 173)

Once again, then, it is not cocaine itself which causes addiction, but a factor in the addict. Indeed, this is a view of addiction which is more advanced than some theories prevalent today.

Furthermore, for Freud cocaine had become an unpredictable object. He noted that in some people, yet not in others, a toxic effect appears, and it is impossible to predict this reaction (Byck 1974: 174). He concludes:

> I suspect that the reason for the irregularity of the cocaine effect lies in the individual variations in excitability and in the variation of the condition of the vasomotor nerves on which cocaine acts. Since little attention has been paid to this factor of individual predisposition, and the degree of excitability generally cannot be known, I consider it advisable to abandon so far as possible subcutaneous injection of cocaine in the treatment of internal and nervous disorders. (Byck 1974: 175)

For Freud, the factor of individual predisposition, the lack of knowledge about the degree of excitability and the consequent unpredictability of the object cocaine, can no longer be reconciled with neurophysiological thinking and the discourse of medical/ pharmacological practice. Indeed, the variable (and still unpredictable) factor of the (pre)-disposition of the subject has completely subverted even the possibility of a medical, neurophysiological approach to an understanding and treatment of mental suffering and addiction.

Having arrived at this impasse in Freud's work on cocaine, we might say that he had stumbled upon the impossible desire of the hysteric.

Conclusion

From this point on, it is clear that Freud's passionate interest in cocaine had 'ceased to write itself'. He had lost his object of fantasy, only to substitute it for another one, which would open different pathways and eventually lead him to the discovery of the unconscious. This object was the desire of the hysteric. It had disrupted his research on cocaine and it would continue to influence the subsequent trajectory of his work, on more than one occasion. A spanner in the works of Freud always seemed to lead to change in a new direction...

In 1888, the year after the last paper on cocaine, Freud published an article on hysteria. I will conclude this chapter with a quotation illustrating the change of direction:

> To begin with, internal medication is to be disrecommended here and narcotic drugs are to be warned against. To prescribe a narcotic drug in an acute hysteria is nothing less than a serious technical mistake. (Freud 1888d: 55)

Notes

[1] A book written by E.M. Thornton (1986) is a striking example of this argument. The author claims that Freud was addicted to cocaine during the period in which he made his fundamental discoveries about the human mind, and that the content of his writings bears a great similarity to the grandiose delusions of cocaine-users.

[2] In this connection I should like to mention the excellent work by Fernando Geberovich, (1984) *Une douleur irresistible;* Sylvie le Poulichet's (1987) *Toxicomanies et Psychanalyse;* Eduardo Vera Ocampo's (1989) *L'envers de la toxicomanie;* and Jean Allouch's (1984) *Lettre pour Lettre.* The chapter entitled 'Freud coquero', in this last book, proved an invaluable source of inspiration for my own reading of Freud's 'Cocaine papers'

FREUD'S STUDIES ON COCAINE

Albrecht Hirschmüller

The cocaine studies

Freud scholarship has evaluated Freud's studies on cocaine in very different ways. Some biographers consider them brilliant and still of relevance to the subject, and celebrate Freud as 'one of the founders of modern psychopharmacology' (Byck 1974: xvii). Some see in Freud's self-experiments with cocaine the roots of his introspective capabilities, and thus emphasise their importance in connection with Freud's self-analysis and theory of dreams.[1] Others stress how Freud failed to recognise the importance of cocaine's local anaesthetic effects, which might have made him world famous. Some have taken the fact that Freud did not himself become addicted to cocaine as evidence of his ego strength (Eissler 1964: 196). Others have claimed that by unreservedly recommending the use of cocaine, Freud was well on the way to becoming a threat to the public.

More recently, however, the cocaine papers have been used to suggest that Freud was not straightforward in the way he presented his findings. They have been used as evidence that Freud tricked his readers, and that his discoveries were 'invented' rather than based on empirical research. In this chapter, then, I propose to reconstruct carefully the historical context of the cocaine papers, in order that we might arrive at a more objective re-evaluation of their significance.

It was on May 21st, 1884, that Freud first mentioned the cocaine project to his fiancée, Martha Bernays. He ordered the drug via a Viennese pharmacy from the Darmstadt producer, E. Merck.[2] A few weeks later the substance was in his hands and he began his experiments.

Over the following days, Freud took cocaine about twelve times, and studied its physical and psychical effects. He soon become convinced of and enthusiastic about 'the wonderful stimulating effects of coca' (Byck 1974: 60). The drug did not produce in him any feeling of being 'altered',[3] but 'exhilaration and lasting euphoria'.

> One senses an increase of self-control and feels more vigorous and more capable of work; on the other hand, if one works, one

> misses the heightening of the mental powers which alcohol, tea or coffee induce. One is simply normal, and soon finds it difficult to believe that one is under the influence of any drug at all. (Byck 1974: 60)

The drug helped Freud overcome irritating bouts of depression, digestive troubles and headaches.

A few days after his first experiment, Freud attempted to make therapeutic use of cocaine by recommending it to a friend, to help wean him from the morphine to which he was addicted. Ernst Fleischl von Marxow was ten years older than Freud, and an assistant to Ernst Brücke at the Physiological Institute of Vienna. Admired and envied by Freud, Fleischl was a talented scientist and gifted experimentalist, a man with a broad interest in art around whom a circle of colleagues from the medical avant-garde of Vienna had gathered.

The story of this famous man's illness is usually told as follows. He had been infected whilst working as an assistant in the Pathological Institute in 1871. Part of his right thumb had been amputated, and he suffered from painful relapsing neuromas. As a result of these he had become severely addicted to morphine.

On the 7th May, 1884, Freud proposed the use of cocaine to Fleischl as a means of withdrawing from morphine. The attempt appeared to be successful—as Freud enthusiastically reported to Martha. Unfortunately the pain soon recurred, and the Fleischl's attempt to withdraw from morphine had to be suspended... However, this story raises many questions, and we shall return to it later.

On June 5th Freud began a study of the scientific literature on cocaine, in order to prepare his own publication. Only two weeks later, he had finished the piece, and it appeared on July 1st in a Viennese periodical. Freud's study is a comprehensive summary of the literature, and describes various possibilities for therapeutic uses of the drug. It also includes a precise description of his experiments, and stresses the value of cocaine in the treatment of the 'morphine habit'. However, if we examine this study more closely, we find traces of the hasty—perhaps even hectic—final phase of its production. Untypically, Freud makes many slips. He miswrites names, confuses places and dates, gives the title of works imprecisely, and even makes a mistake in the formula for cocaine.

Without doubt, Freud's evaluation of the literature on cocaine was biased. He denounced the warnings he encountered against use of the drug as slanderous reports. He was also uncritical in his acceptance of enthusiastic reports he found in the *Therapeutic Gazette* from Detroit, despite the very dubious scientific reputation of this periodical.

Freud's study evoked little interest. During a medical congress at Copenhagen in June of that year, Heinrich Obersteiner gave a report on Freud's use of cocaine as a means of treating morphine addiction (Obersteiner 1886). However, discussion at the congress focused on other issues. Indeed, Freud himself seemed to lose interest in cocaine during the summer. He began to doubt the value of his findings, and turned to other scientific interests. But on returning from his holiday in October, he learned that the discovery of cocaine as a local anaesthetic for the eye had—meanwhile—spread throughout the world. There is little doubt that he regretted it was the name of his friend Karl Koller, and not is own, which was on everybody's lips. At the end of October he wrote to Minna Bernays that '[c]ocaine has brought me a great deal of credit, but the lion's share has gone elsewhere' (Jones 1953: 98).

Meanwhile, Fleischl had developed close contacts with Merck, the cocaine manufacturer. Fleischl's high consumption of cocaine had been noted. As is shown by the firm's books, at this time Fleischl was ordering his cocaine directly through the Institute of Physiology.[4]

As a consequence of these contacts, the company suggested to Freud that he might research the properties of *ecgonin*, an alkaloid derived from cocaine. Merck's offered to finance the project, and Freud accepted.

As part of his investigation, Freud considered how he could study objectively changes in body strength and reaction time under the influence of the drug. Ecgonin itself did not appear to have any significant effect as a drug, but Freud's methods seemed to show a great deal concerning the general physiological effects of cocaine. It was this investigation, then, which formed the basis of Freud's second cocaine study.

To assess his body strength whilst under the influence of the drug, Freud used two different dynamometers.[5] In his attempt to establish a baseline for his experiments, Freud discovered marked differences in the degree of his body strength from one day to another. He also discovered a certain periodicity *during* the day, with 'downs' in the early morning and late evening, and 'ups' from noon to the early afternoon. These 'biorhythms' have now been established and documented in connection with a number of significant parameters in plant and animal physiology.[6]

In self-experiments, Freud discovered that cocaine increased the strength of his grip by several kilograms, and that this effect ran parallel with the degree of euphoria induced by the drug. His results appeared during January 1885, in the *Weiner Medizinische Wochenschrift*. This article remained Freud's only experimental psychophysiological study. Despite working without a sophisticated methodology, and without a fully equipped psychophysiological laboratory, Freud had nevertheless produced results of much more than marginal importance. Indeed, we might suppose that he would have arrived at even more valuable findings had he continued to work in this field.

Debacles

On March 5th, 1885, Freud delivered a lecture to the Psychiatric Society of Vienna. He presented a summary of his published work on cocaine. He also stressed the value of cocaine to psychiatry, as a stimulant for psychical weakness and depression, and as a valuable therapeutic aid in the treatment of withdrawal from morphine. The only significant development in Freud's views on cocaine was that he now began to recommend subcutaneous injections of the drug:

> On the basis of my experiences with the effects of cocaine, I have no hesitation in recommending the administration of cocaine for such withdrawal cures in subcutaneous injections of 0.03-0.05g per dose, without any fear of increasing the dose. (Byck 1974: 117)

Freud never quoted from this lecture in future years, and neither did he include it in his summary of his publications (Freud 1897b), nor in the separate collection of works on organic neurology (Brun 1936). Siegfried Bernfeld, in an impressive study, has pointed out that this should be interpreted as a slip, indicating that Freud's recommendation of cocaine injections for morphine addiction later aroused feelings of guilt and shame in him. Indeed, Freud admitted as much in *The Interpretation of Dreams*.[7]

In December 1884 a report on Freud's cocaine studies appeared in the *St Louis Medical and Surgical Journal* (Pollak 1884). Freud had become well-known as an expert on cocaine—even as far as America—and had received requests to send cocaine to the United States. Liquid extracts of cocaine, of a rather dubious quality, were available on the American market. The cocaine produced by Parke, Davis & Co. of Detroit was of this ilk, and seems to have been less reliable than the preparation used by Freud from E. Merck.

Parke-Davis, therefore, were eager to have a respectable scientist prove the quality of their product. It was Freud who undertook this investigation on their behalf, for which he was offered a honorarium of 60 Gulden, in April 1885. Freud's expert opinion was published in August, in the context of an article by Gutt, who alleged that Merck's cocaine was over-priced and rarely available, and who openly advertised Parke cocaine. The Merck company duly protested, complaining that the article was 'a publication in favour of an American firm in the disguise of a study of scientific value' (Freud 1885a: col. 1036).

Meanwhile, personal relations between Freud and Fleischl had intensified. Fleischl's condition had become a cause for concern, and Freud joined him during sleepless nights of confusion and excitement.

By the end of May 1885 it became clear to Freud that Fleischl was deeply drug-dependent, spent a fortune on cocaine, and took morphine in doses which sometimes caused him to fall into severe delirium. For weeks, Breuer, Exner and Freud took turns to stay with Fleischl overnight, during which he underwent states of unconsciousness, sleeplessness, and seizures with cramps and anxiety (Israëls 1993: 228-230). When Freud returned from Paris in the spring of the following year, Fleischl's condition had deteriorated even further. He had been unable to withdraw from morphine, but had instead developed a morphine-cocaine dependency with severe complications. In 1892 he died. A letter from Breuer describes powerfully the last, painful day in the life of this formerly great scientist.

Was the way in which Freud approached Fleischl's case a 'quack treatment'? Is one justified in describing Freud as a 'liar and scientific charlatan' who attempted to hoax the public?[8] We should remind ourselves that, in Freud's day, addiction was not viewed as a disease in its own right, and the drawing of a distinction between detoxification and the treatment of addiction was unusual. In Freud's eyes, the use of cocaine to facilitate withdrawal from morphine had been successful; Fleischl had indeed survived for 10 or 11 days without morphine. It was only his pain and the necessity of another operation which had driven him back to morphine again. Freud viewed the deterioration of Fleischl's condition as a consequence of the physical pain from which he suffered, leaving him dependent upon analgesics. In my opinion, there is no question of Freud attempting to deliberately mislead in his version of events, as Israëls and Busse suggest. However, it is clear that Freud placed himself in a complicated and conflictual situation, and this can be detected in his publications on cocaine.

Alternative reasons for the brief success of Freud's treatment can—perhaps—also be inferred from the personality structure of the patient. This was the approach taken by Haas in 1983. Haas argued that it would be short-sighted to regard Fleischl as a man in pain with drug-dependency as a secondary problem. Instead, Haas argues, Fleischl suffered from polytoxicomania and—like many drug-addicts—was able to hide this completely from everyone around him, including Freud. Indeed, some recently discovered details from the family history and biography of Fleischl seem to support this view.[9]

Re-assessments

At the same time as Freud began to recognise the seriousness of Fleischl's condition, the first article stressing the dangers of cocaine was published.

Albrecht Erlenmeyer wrote that cocaine addiction had joined alcoholism and morphine addiction as a 'third scourge of humanity'.[10] He likened the attempt to substitute morphine with cocaine with efforts to drive out the devil by Beelzebub.

In his last cocaine study of 1887, Freud admitted that the value of cocaine for morphine addicts had been annihilated by the fact that they simply tended to become dependent upon cocaine in addition to morphine. However, Freud insisted that cocaine did on take any victims entirely on its own account, and reproached Erlenmeyer with having made grave errors in his reports. Freud's opinion was shared by other scientific authorities, such as Obersteiner.

Thereafter, Freud continued to take cocaine from time to time, in order to fight his own depressive states. He appreciated its stimulating effects; he used it to loosen his tongue when he was invited to the house of Charcot in Paris. Indeed, he continued to prescribe it freely to friends and members of his family.

Cocaine was far from being abandoned, despite Erlenmeyer's attack. This is shown clearly by the thriving market in paramedical products at the time. Numerous tonics, elixirs, syrups and nerve-stimulants contained—variously—opium, arsenic, alcohol, chloroform and bromides. In addition to these were many cocaine preparations, and food and drinks containing cocaine.

In Atlanta, Georgia, 1885, John Pemberton produced a wine containing coca. One year later he removed the alcohol, added an extract of cola, and called the product *Coca-Cola*. It was not until 1906 that the Food and Drug Act forced the company to remove cocaine from the Coca-Cola formula.[11]

Pemberton had in fact been preceded, by Angelo Mariani in Paris. From 1885 he produced a coca wine, *Vin Mariani*. Numerous famous figures of the time wrote enthusiastically about this drink, and endorsed it strongly. From 1895, Mariani published albums with letters of recommendation from people such as Thomas Edison, H.G. Wells, Henrik Ibsen, Henri Poincaré, Auguste Rodin, Emile Zola and Pope Leo XIII (Eyguesier 1983).

Cocaine was in great demand and became a drug '*en vogue*' among artists and writers. Stevenson's *Dr. Jekyll and Mr. Hyde* (1885) is possibly the most famous example of a book composed under the influence of cocaine (Grinspoon & Bakalar 1976: 27). Sherlock Holmes was prescribed cocaine by Dr. Watson in 'The Sign of the Four' (1890): Arthur Conan Doyle had become acquainted with the drug in his ophthalmological practice (Grinspoon & Bakalar 1976: 36). Even in the 1920s, cocaine was still the subject of avant-garde literature. Jean Cocteau, Max Brod, Gottfried Benn, and others, have described its effects.

Conclusion

On the relevance of the cocaine studies to Freud's other work, Haas writes:

> From our contemporary point of view the cocaine studies, together with the fiancée letters, are something of an embryological nodal point, containing the most important structures and *primordia* of Freud's later works. In the passages on the history of the coca cultus, we see already Freud's interest in the topic of a father religion. The multiple therapeutic possibilities of the drug may be seen as a precursor of the trend according to which he would later regard psychoanalysis as the single therapeutic tool for a whole host of illnesses. His self-experiments with cocaine, and his admirable faculty of self-insight, perhaps show Freud already on the way to self-analysis. And finally we

see his capability to stand decisively for a conviction, and not to give it up when attacked, neglected, or isolated. (Haas 1983: 172)

Indeed, the cocaine papers demonstrate that Freud was a scientist with curiosity and intuition, who took his own observations so seriously that he could not rest until he had found explanations for them. They show that Freud was a man who was used to relying more upon his own experience than upon the scientific literature he read—and who was often justified in doing so. They show Freud as a young doctor, eager to advance quickly by his scientific work, and consequently in danger of jumping too quickly to conclusions, rather than grounding his theories through more reserved and patient scientific work. Freud's works on cocaine also show that he used the drug without prejudice, and took the risk of ignoring critical and cautious warnings.

Evidently, Freud did not fully appreciate the problems of addiction. One reason for this blind-spot may have been his own personality. For although Freud himself did not develop cocaine dependency, curiously however, he was singularly unable to give up smoking. The same man who had abandoned his ideas on the therapeutic possibilities of an addictive drug, would nevertheless attest freely in his later years that he owed at least a portion of his creativity to his cigar.

Notes

[1] See, for instance, Vom Scheidt 1973a, 1973b; Schott 1986.

[2] Merck 1883-86: entry of 24th April, 1884. See also Hirschmüller 1995b.

[3] *'Alterationsgefühl'* in the original. Byck 1974 has 'feeling of excitement', which is certainly not a good translation.

[4] Merck 1883-86: entry of 31st April, 1884. See also Hirschmüller 1995b.

[5] See Hirschmüller 1995a for details.

[6] See Luce 1971.

[7] See Bernfeld 1953; Byck 1974: 347-352; Freud 1900 (in particular the dream of Irma's injection, the dream of the botanical monograph, and the *'non vixit'* dream); Vom Scheidt 1973b; Haas 1983.

[8] For such as assessment of Freud, see Busse 1993: 52, 54, a review of Israëls 1993.

[9] See Haas 1983.

[10] *'Dritte Geißel der Menschiet'* in the original.

[11] See Andrews & Solomon 1975: 10-12; Kahn 1960: 55ff.

IN THE BEGINNING OF PSYCHOANALYSIS THERE WAS EUPHORIA

Pierre Eyguesier

Introduction

Why such a provocative title?

Perhaps one might expect something more along the lines of 'in the beginning there was *hysteria*', or 'the *symptom*', or '*discontent* within our civilisation'. As this paper is a reading of Freud's involvement with cocaine, one might suspect that the 'euphoria' refers to the effect produced by the drug. But given the devastation caused by abuse of drugs such as cocaine, perhaps this 'euphoria' appears a little *suspicious*...

Indeed, situating the 'beginning' of psychoanalysis in what is commonly called Freud's 'cocaine episode' perhaps appears equally dubious. After all, commentators seem to agree that this phase was a 'lateral interest', an 'allotrion',[1] a sort of hobby which Freud soon cast aside in order to concentrate on more serious matters—such as hypnosis, the cathartic method and, eventually, psychoanalysis itself. So even if one were led to believe that the cocaine episode was important, raising it to the status of the 'beginning' of psychoanalysis might be regarded as an extravagance, characteristic of commentators who are obsessed with origins. Incessantly these commentators search for the sources of the Nile of psychoanalysis. At one moment these sources will be the genius of Freud himself, at another the risk he took in occupying himself with hysterical patients whom medicine was unable to treat, or—at yet another moment—his auto-analysis, or one of many other kinds of explanation.

To return to 'euphoria': there is nothing less 'euphoric' than the suffering which inspired psychoanalysis as a novel answer to our civilisation and its discontents. Nor is euphoria what we should expect from analysis which, at best, allows the patient to attain 'ordinary misery'. Analysis is decidedly not a means of access to beatitude, nor to the rather inane happiness which is most commonly connoted by the word 'euphoria'. Has a patient ever floated on clouds of happiness on the completion of analysis? Indeed, I can anticipate the reservations of the Lacanians, in whose view the completion of analysis is synonymous with 'desubjectivation' (*desêtre*). From this perspective, even if a 'removal of the repression' occurred it would certainly not be accompanied with 'euphoria'. Euphoria would denote, rather, that the subject had pierced the screen of fantasy.

In what follows I attempt to show how I arrived at the notion that Freud embarked upon the psychoanalytic voyage of discovery—as it were—under the influence of cocaine. Freud called it a 'magical substance'—a locution which, I shall argue, should be interpreted as '*talking* substance'. I will also show how, in our day and age, long after Freud awoke from the dreams into which cocaine had plunged him, his encounter with the drug enables us to revive a dimension of psychoanalysis which has been consigned to oblivion. Ever since the psychoanalytic religion became the opium of the analytic community, the dimension of laughing, gaiety—of *desire* in its rawest aspect—has been neglected. In short, it is Spinoza's notion of 'joy' to which I referring, which he placed at the pinnacle of human virtues.

In the beginning

I shall not dwell upon the various theories concerning the inception of psychoanalysis. In my view, the problem with most of these is that they lend to Freud's progressive development the aspect of necessity, which—quite evidently—is only applicable retroactively.

Furthermore, if a theology has grown up around Freud's work then a description of the master's itinerary has become a matter for hagiographers. I am referring, for instance, to Ernest Jones's excessive rhetoric on the subject of self-analysis, which is taken as the starting-point of the discovery of the 'abysmal depths of the unconscious' (Jones 1953: 351-60). There are, however, other approaches, which do not regard Freud's 'genius' or 'Judaism' as necessary conditions for his discovery of the unconscious. More appropriately, its discovery is attributed to the hysterical patients themselves, with Freud as the 'sufficient condition' whose discourse has to be interpreted as 'a simple partitioning of the discourse of the Other' (Nassif 1977: 637).

Once we adopt this point of view, it becomes possible to reinterpret the historical events entwined with the psychoanalytic voyage of discovery in the same way as the Stoics regarded fate: that is, as a sequence of 'quasi-causes' upon which Man could have no effect whatsoever. Paradoxically, Man's 'liberty' consisted in following the events as they presented themselves to him.

In this light, the cocaine episode betokens an event of far-reaching significance for our understanding of what is meant by 'Freudian orientation'. To the best of my knowledge, it has never been fully recognised as such. 'Freudian orientation' should be understood here not only in its 'cardinal' sense, as an orientation taken up for the first time *by Freud,* in the direction of the field of 'functional troubles', a concept which is the precursor of neurosis. It should also be understood in a figurative sense—that is, as the shaping of a *style,* of a particular way of proceeding which foreshadowed what was yet to come. Finally, on the outskirts of the great psychoanalytic oeuvre, 'Freudian orientation' refers to an Orient, an imaginary, which can be rediscovered at a profit.

Without further preliminaries, I present an excerpt from a book I wrote twelve years ago, which concerns the 'right encounter' (or 'τυχη', to follow the Aristotelian term honoured by Lacan) between Freud and cocaine:

> In 1884 ... Freud devoted much time and effort to what we would today describe as 'fundamental research'. However, the praiseworthy results he achieved did not prevent him from casting sidelong glances at the possibility of more lucrative occupations, which his standing as a physician could not offer. It was not that Freud was uninterested in providing therapeutic care for his patients. His dedicated intervention at the bedside of a hysterical patient, and his manifest worries at seeing his discipline (neurology) misused where the application of therapy was concerned, are evidence for this. In the words of his biographers, Freud simply nurtured 'other ambitions'. Parallel with these uncertainties, Freud was plagued by more personal problems. He had been engaged for several years, and was waiting impatiently to establish himself in order to get married. In addition to this his closest friend and colleague, Ernst von Fleischl-Marxow, had suffered a serious, painful injury, and had become addicted to morphine through habitual use of the drug as a pain-killer. Taken by themselves, these factors might shed some light on why Freud complained of various disorders—cardiac, digestive, and others—which he described as the effect of 'neurasthenia'.
>
> It was against this background, then, that Freud accidentally came across an article in which the properties of a remarkable drug were described... Limiting myself to what might have cap-

> tured Freud's attention, the physicians maintained that coca and its derivatives enabled decisive success in the cure of disorders such as neurasthenia, hypochondria, functional digestive and functional cardiac disorders, as well as in the treatment of morphine poisoning.
>
> ...One can easily surmise the extent to which this discovery must have spoken to Freud's imagination. The encounter with cocaine was thus a radical 'effect of fortune' for Freud, as a man suffering from neurasthenia, cardiac and digestive troubles, a physician confronted with hysterical patients, a neurologist plagued by uncertainty and doubts about the therapeutic effectiveness of his discipline, a researcher with uncertain prospects, and—finally—as someone whose best friend was a morphine addict. (Eyguesier 1983)

The magical cure

When one examines the various traces of this episode, one is confronted with a marriage of—firstly—the effects of cocaine on Freud (who conducted his experiments with cocaine largely upon himself) and—secondly—scientific work.

In order that we might survey the influence of cocaine on Freud, I shall attempt a succinct itemisation of the effects produced by the drug.

(1) Cocaine acts like a potion, making one 'talkative':

> The bit of cocaine I have just taken is making me talkative, my little woman... Here I am, making silly confessions to you, my sweet darling, and really without any reason whatever unless it is the cocaine that makes me talk so much. (Letter to Martha Bernays, Byck 1974: 164)

(2) Cocaine acts like a love potion:

> Woe to you, my Princess, when I come. I will kiss you quite red and feed you till you are plump. And if you are forward you shall see who is the stronger, a gentle little girl who doesn't eat enough or a big wild man *who has cocaine in his body*. (Letter to Martha Bernays, Byck 1974: 10)

(3) Cocaine facilitates 'the disappearance of elements in one's general state of well-being which cause depression' (Byck 1974: 60), concerning which Freud later wrote:

> In neurosis, then, great attention is paid... perhaps because the subject-matter of such ideas fits in with the mood of the neurosis, or perhaps because antithetic ideas, which could otherwise have been absent, flourish in the soil of a neurosis. (Freud 1892-93: 121-122)

(4) Cocaine 'removes repression'. Because the notion of repression had not at this time been formulated by Freud, one might be disinclined to accept this conceptual anachronism. However, in my view this notion allows one to account for the way in which a euphoric state appears to supplant a feeling of unease (or, more accurately, a *neurasthenic* state) under the influence of cocaine. It was in these same terms that Freud described the effect of cocaine upon his own ailments:

> If one takes a minimally active dose... while in excellent health and does not expect any special exertion thereafter, one can hardly perceive any surprising effect. It is different, however, if this dose of cocaine hydrochloride is taken by a subject whose general health is impaired by fatigue or hunger. After a short time... he feels as though he had been raised to the full height of intellectual and bodily vigour, in a state of euphoria, which is distinguished from the euphoria after consumption of alcohol by the absence of any feeling of alteration. However astonishing this effect of ingestion of coca may be, the absence of signs that could distinguish the state from the normal euphoria of good health makes it even more likely that we will underestimate it. As soon as the contrast between the present state and the state before the ingestion of cocaine is forgotten, it is difficult to believe that one is under the influence of a foreign agent... (Byck 1974: 114)

It seems to me that this passage is of crucial importance. This 'effect of contrast', described here by Freud, is nothing less than the conceptual precursor of a 'removal of repression'. The effect of cocaine demonstrates that desire is 'split': one can clearly distinguish between a compartmentalised before and after, for as soon as the euphoric state emerges one forgets one's previous state. However, it should be emphasised that the 'new' state is no different from how we feel normally. Here a striking paradox comes to light: the 'better' state which one obtains through cocaine was, in fact, 'already there'—or, more precisely, it *is* 'already there', biding its time and awaiting the moment to surface.

Likewise, Freud would later observe that under hypnosis his hysterical patients expressed themselves in a 'normal fashion, simply normal', and would maintain that psychoanalysis does not equip the patient with an extra 'advantage' but—like cocaine—merely enables him to reach the stage of a *normal* 'more cheerful mood' (Byck 1974: 104):

> The psychic effect of cocaïnum muriaticum in doses of 0.05-0.10g consists of exhilaration and lasting euphoria, which does not differ in any way from the normal euphoria... One is simply normal. (Byck 1974: 60)

In other words, for Freud normality was tantamount to euphoria. It is as though having just discovered an artifice which allowed what had become unconscious to surface, he immediately declared its non-specificity. This aspect of cocaine—the way in which it does not produce an effect different from a normal state of mind—was what Freud endeavoured to conceptualise, in different ways, in his scientific writings on the drug.

Freud systematically recorded the effects of cocaine on his 'symptoms' by testing them scientifically against the knowledge passed on to him by his professors. He equipped himself with a dynamometer and Exner's neuro-amoebimeter, and attempted to measure the variations of the 'psychical reaction time or of muscular force' after an intake of cocaine. Clearly, Wundt's ideal underlies and informs Freud's efforts, and Meynert's conception of the brain is easily traceable in Freud's description of the euphoric state as 'a well-nourished cerebral cortex which "is not conscious" of the organs of the body to which it belongs' (Byck 1974: 61). Furthermore, in order to explain why cocaine provides surplus energy—allegedly the reason why Peruvian *coqueros* survived a famine by taking the drug—Freud evokes the 'principle of constancy' which formed the bedrock of thermodynamics, a cutting-edge experimental science at the time.

However, what Freud strove to emphasise was the *psychical influence* of the drug. This prompted him to separate its effects into 'direct' and 'indirect' action:

> I do not consider the cocaine action itself to be a direct one—possibly on the motor-nerve substance or on the muscles—but indirect, effected by an improvement of the general state of well-being. (Byck 1974: 102)

In short, cocaine's properties were not of a pharmacological nature at all, but rested on their capacity to alter the general humour *via* an increase of 'muscular energy':

> It became clear to me that the above-mentioned variation in motor-power, which does not depend on the time of day is an expression of the general state of well-being; after all, the subjective phenomenon of this state as bodily feeling (*Gemeingefühl* [coenesthesia]) and mood is to a great extent associated with motor efficiency. (Byck 1974: 102)

Elsewhere Freud wrote:

> In this connection one might recall the fact that the human nervous system has an undoubted, if somewhat obscure, influence on the nourishment of tissues; psychological factors can, after all, cause a healthy man to lose weight. (Byck 1974: 69).

What prompted me to undertake more research in this area was the fact that Freud conceived this 'obscure' influence of 'psychological factors' upon the body entirely in terms of *energy*, rather than as an effect of *language*. Freud drew no conclusions from the effects of cocaine upon the motor aspect of language; his investigation of the drug fails to take into account its pharmacological effects *alongside* its capacity for activating the 'speech engine'.

The scholar's dust and the sorcerer's page

Freud drew no distinction between the euphoria induced by coca, and the euphoria of 'normal well-being'. It simply corresponds to the state of 'feeling well'. Furthermore, the fact that this effect is linked with his 'idiosyncrasy' did not elude Freud's observation. Indeed, he used it as a defence against the accusations levelled against him when it became obvious cocaine was addictive.

The euphoria of cocaine corresponds to a number of its attested effects: on digestion, respiration, 'functional sexual disorders', the voice, and the gaze. I propose to take a closer look at these zones affected by cocaine. I intend to do this by immersing the question of the psychological influence in a wider context. From the beginning of his researches, and after having given up hope of becoming the discoverer of the anaesthetic features of the drug, Freud consulted the existing literature on cocaine, and read many accounts of the various uses to which the drug had been put, all of which seemed to corroborate his hypotheses. For instance, in the works of Mantegazza and Hammond he encountered results of experiments establishing the medical virtues of the drug in cases as diverse as asthma, dyspepsia, melancholia, nausea, vomiting, hysteria and vaginismus. I shall provide only one quotation from this series of communications, which illustrates the lesson Freud drew from them. Mantegazza reports:

> In the same conditions, after the excitation of salivation, a dryness of the pituitary of the eyes occurs, while the orgasm takes place in the genital apparatus. Besides, this phenomenon was already familiar to the Indians from time immemorial, for their Venus was represented holding a coca leaf in her hand. (Mariani 1895: chapter 1)

In Freud we find the following:

> The natives of South America, who represented their goddess of love with coca leaves in her hand, did not doubt the stimulative effect of coca on the genitalia. Mantegazza confirms that the *coqueros* sustain a high degree of potency right into old age; he even reports cases of the restoration of potency and the disappearance of functional weakness following the use of coca. (Byck 1974: 73)

However, one source of writings on cocaine of which Freud could not have been aware was that surrounding the consumption, in France, of *coca wine*. The wine was produced by Mariani, a rather mysterious character, who was regarded by his contemporaries as much more than a simple merchant. In a publicity stunt clearly ahead of its time, Mariani invited prominent 'contemporary figures'—all of whom gladly accepted—to contribute a drawing, poem, or epigram in praise of coca wine. The 'albums' in which these were collected and published are true repositories of celebrities from the end of the nineteenth century.[2]

However, beyond their undeniably publicity-oriented function, these albums seem to betoken the launch of a new symbol of desire. Coca wine—the albums fervently attest—leads to action, and simultaneously induces people to talk. These two effects cannot be dissociated. The drug is a panacea: for some it sharpens the gaze, for some it strengthens the voice, and for others it enhances eloquence. Not least, a great many of those who drank it associated coca wine with sexual desire. This association was sometimes made in a straightforward and graphic fashion—indeed, a *very* graphic fashion: I was surprised to come across one of the 'darker horses' of Mariani's albums, in which some contributions were considered too explicit for public circulation.

This was probably the last 'panacea' to sweep Europe before the dawn of scientific medicine, which tolled the death-knell for all curative potions based on alcohol, opium and coca. Afterwards, production of medicine would be placed exclusively in the hands of pharmaceutical companies, controlled by the state. As the final panacea, and the final 'talking drug', Mariani's coca wine furnishes us with the means of apprehending what Freud conceived of as the psychical influence of cocaine.

The way in which coca—in its different forms—occupies the place of 'phallus' allows us to understand not only Freud's enthusiasm and his wish to write 'a poem in its praise', but also the odd fact that coca put into perspective for Freud the pulsational objects which—in accordance with Lacan's theory—are 'the causes of desire'. These include the voice, the gaze, hence nothing speech-like. An account of the magical powers of cocaine is now possible, which makes use of Freud's topographical, economical, functional and mnemic categories. To this end one should take seriously the hypothesis that, during the belle époque at the end of the nineteenth century, which witnessed the rise of an increasing malaise in society, coca was a natural element that could be elevated metaphorically to the rank of 'signifier of desire'. If we add to this the figure of a sorcerer, then all the ingredients are in place for a magical cure, the analysis of which involves in a certain way the properties of cocaine.

Medical and pharmacological accounts of psychotropic effects examine direct repercussions on the chemistry of the brain, and overlook the fact that drugs can also *speak*. An important lesson can be drawn from the cocaine episode, then. It was because Freud interpreted the chemical signs of cocaine (on the 'nervous substratum') *only with the help of other signs* that the drug had only a tempered effect upon him. These other signs were his expectations as a 'man of devotion and subject of absolute knowledge'. This is also the reason why, after the devastating effects of the use of cocaine had been uncovered and denounced, Freud was able to content himself with the effects of speech, with the magical powers (for the word 'magic' is often used by Freud, and deserves to be emphasised) with which words are endowed. Instead of his *pharmakon*, he explored the effects of speech and magic—that is, the magical powers of words.

More than ten years after publishing a full-length work on this subject (Eyguesier 1983), I persist in thinking that this episode is worthy of disinterment from the pre-analytic underground in which it is buried. It represents a first encounter for Freud with the chaos of functional disorders, from which—after his stay in Paris—he would produce his teachings on hysteria and neurasthenia. It also marks the first collusion between the subject of desire and the scientific subject, vividly illustrating how Freud participates *as a subject* in his scientific endeavour to push back the boundaries of knowledge. The episode demonstrates the marriage between science and poetry.

In addition, this allotrion lent to the beginnings of psychoanalysis a genuine touch of euphoria—a normal euphoria, indistinguishable from the drug-induced variety. Sadly, however, this dimension seems to have been lost from the heredity of psychoanalysis.

Notes

1 αλλοτριον: 'allotrion', or 'an other way'.

2 Editions of these albums, containing the original consignments of solicited personalities, as well as some 'censored' from publication, have been deposited in the National Library in Paris, by Mariani's heirs.

FRANZ BRENTANO, FREUD'S PHILOSOPHICAL MENTOR

Aviva Cohen

Introduction

During his time at the University of Vienna, Freud attended a series of lectures by the philosopher Franz Brentano. In this paper, I will argue that Brentano's philosophy influenced Freud's work to a significant degree. I shall focus upon Brentano's early text, *Psychology from an Empirical Standpoint*, in particular the account of 'judgement' he develops in this work.

Brentano asserted that every mental act has, within it, an object, although there are different ways in which thoughts may be directed towards their 'immanent' object. This, his 'intentionality thesis', marks the difference between mental phenomena and physical phenomena. Brentano claims that we are immediately certain of the 'reality' of an 'inner perception', and that our knowledge of 'external' truths is—in contrast—by means of secondary mechanisms.

I will argue that Freud uses Brentanian principles in his discussion of the distinction between ideas and 'reality' in his 'A Project for a Scientific Psychology', and in several of his metapsychological papers. Also, I will suggest that it was Brentano's theory of judgement which eventually enabled Freud to repudiate his 'seduction theory', which dealt with the question of external 'reality' and the 'truth' attributable to an object of thought. We encounter some of these issues expressed in a more mature form in Freud's 1925 essay 'On Negation', where his discussion of affirmation and denial is—I maintain—drawn directly from Brentano's early theory of judgement and his intentionality thesis in general.

Historical connections

Freud enrolled at the University of Vienna in 1873. By this time, medical students were no longer required to attend lectures in philosophy. However, Freud elected to do just that. During the winter term of 1874 he joined a weekly seminar, given by the recently appointed Professor of Philosophy, Franz Brentano.

Many enthusiastic students would publish descriptions of these lectures. Their reports depict Brentano as a striking and charismatic figure, whose impact on the lives of his students was dramatic. He is said to have inspired lasting and contemplative devotion to 'truth', 'philosophy' and his own, 'otherworldly' presence (McAlister 1976: 6). Time after time he received tributes from former students—for example, Edmund Husserl, who wrote that

> I was vacillating between studying in mathematics and devoting my life to philosophy, Brentano's lectures were the deciding factor. (McAlister 1976: 47)

There is a great deal of evidence to suggest that Brentano's philosophical and psychological teachings had a significant impact of Freud's theoretical development. Since the publication of Freud's letters to Eduard Silberstein[1] it has been possible to correct many of the oversights and inaccuracies which have frequently clouded Freud scholarship in this area.

We can, for example, revise the common notion that Freud was unsympathetic towards philosophy. I do not intend to discuss this in great detail, but shall suggest one reason for the confusion. It is evident that Freud frequently criticises something he calls 'philosophy'. However, when he does so, he is not referring to the entire discipline, but is following Brentano in a rejection of the speculative metaphysics of Hegel, Shelling and Fichte. Brentano considered himself a natural scientist, working objectively with experience as his guide. He insisted that 'the true method of philosophy is none other than that of natural science'.[2] For Carl Strumpf, among others, 'it was a new, incomparably deeper and more serious way of understanding philosophy' (McAlister 1976: 11).

Freud should be read in this light. He is not referring the work of Brentano when he rails against philosophy. As Peter Gay puts it: 'Freud gave "philosophy" a special meaning. In true Enlightenment fashion, he designated the philosophising of metaphysicians as unhelpful abstractions' (Gay 1988: 119).

However, this is not to deny that Freud provides us with numerous opportunities for misunderstanding. For example, in a letter from Freud to Werner Achelis we read: 'I not only have no capability for philosophy but also no respect for it'. This seems straightforward enough, but further on in the same letter Freud confides:

> in secret, I cannot say this aloud, I believe that metaphysics will one day be seen as a nuisance, as a misuse of thought, as a survival from the period of religious world view, and it will be judged thus. (Freud 1960a: letter of 30th January, 1927)

Freud did not consider his professor a speculative 'metaphysician' in this sense. On the contrary, in a letter of 1875 he refers to Brentano as a

> remarkable man (a believer, a teleologist (!) and a Darwinian, and a damned clever fellow, a genius in fact), who is, in many respects, an ideal human being. (Freud 1989b: 95)

Unfortunately, however, successive Freud biographers have failed to recognise the full significance of this student-teacher relationship. Ernest Jones, for example, claims that Freud took merely a 'passing glance' at Brentano's reading seminars (Jones 1953: 41). Both Freud's correspondence, and the University records, inform us that Freud was, in fact, 'glancing' at philosophy up to three times per week between the winter of 1874 and the end of the summer semester in 1876. It is also worth taking note of a fact which Jones neglects to mention, that Brentano's seminars 'were the only non-medical courses taken by Freud during his whole course of studies (eight semesters)' (Merlan 1949: 451).

It seems we should agree with William J. McGrath's conclusion that 'Jones seriously underestimates Brentano's influence, for as this and many subsequent letters reveal, it was the course with Franz Brentano that most excited Freud during that semester' (McGrath 1986: 101).

Peter Gay is not without his shortcomings on this point. He acknowledges something of Brentano's impact on Freud when he writes that 'Brentano had stimulated and complicated Freud's thinking, and his psychological writings left significant deposits in Freud's mind' (Gay 1988: 29); nevertheless, Gay makes a mistake in the details of his biography which undermines the significance of Freud's relationship to Brentano, and leads Gay to the erroneous conclusion that the influence of Brentano steadily faded into the background.[3]

In this regard, it is also important to note that Freud had been a fervent materialist, carefully planning a winter of study with the leaders of this field in Berlin. At the beginning of 1875 he informs his young friend Silberstein, 'I am as happy as a child at the thought and could not bear the idea of giving up the project' (Freud 1989b: letter of 24th January, 1875). However, just two months later he cancelled his trip and wrote again, this time to declare that he was 'no longer a materialist' and had decided to remain in Vienna. The reason for this decision was that he wished to maintain contact with Brentano. He wrote:

> Especially under Brentano's influence the determination has ripened within me to pursue a Ph.D. in Philosophy and Zoology. Further negotiations are in progress to bring about my enrolment in the philosophy faculty either next semester or nest year. (Freud 1960a: letter of 7th March, 1875)

Freud's enthusiasm for his teacher led him to pursue philosophical studies both in the lecture halls and through conversations in Brentano's home. We can appreciate the intensity of his interest from the following passage, taken from another letter to Silberstein. He writes:

> In short, Brentano cannot possibly be refuted before one has heard and studied him and plundered his stores of knowledge. So sharp a dialectician requires one to hone one's own wits on his before challenging him. (Freud 1960a: letter of 27th March, 1875)

This is a strange comment to make regarding someone who was at this time—supposedly—'fading into the background'.

Theoretical conclusions

I shall now turn to Brentano's theories, and consider the extent to which they informed Freud's thinking. In presenting Brentano's philosophy I will refer only to his early theories, most of which were published in *Psychology from an Empirical Standpoint* in 1874, the same year in which Freud attended first attended his seminar. As we proceed, it may be useful to bear in mind James Barclay's comment that:

> When the philosophical terminology of Brentano and the mechanistic terminology of Freud are stripped from the concept, it

> appears that the essential features of the doctrine of intentionality are found in both systems. (Barclay 1964: 29)

In *Psychology from an Empirical Standpoint*, Brentano searches for characteristics which allow him to identify a class of phenomena exclusive to psychology. The most important of these, he suggests, is *intentional inexistence*—a property common to all mental phenomena but lacking in every physical phenomenon. Similarly, in 'Instincts and Their Vicissitudes' Freud claims to have 'obtained the material necessary for distinguishing between instinctual [drive] stimuli and other (psychological) stimuli that operate on the mind' (Freud 1915a: 118). We will see that his view of the distinction and interaction between the psychical and the physical are analogous to Brentano's teachings.

The lineaments of Brentano's position are expressed most clearly in this famous passage, taken from his *Psychology*:

> Every mental phenomenon is characterised by what the Scholastics of the Middle Ages called the intentional (or mental) in-existence of an object, and what we might call, though not wholly unambiguously, reference to a content, direction towards an object (which is not to be understood here as meaning a thing), or immanent objectivity. Every mental phenomenon includes some thing as object within itself, although they do not all do so in the same way. In presentation something is presented, in judgement something is affirmed or denied, in love loved, in hate hated, in desire desired and so on. (Brentano 1973a: 88)

'Presentation' (*Vorstellung*), judgement (*Urteil*), and 'love/hate' (*Gemutsbewegungen*)—the latter often referred to as 'emotion', 'desire' or 'feeling'—these are the three classes of mental phenomena distinguished in Brentano's account. Each one represents a mental act which refers to its object in a different way. The emphasis is always on the notion of 'activity'. He writes: 'by presentation I do not mean that which is presented, but rather the act of presentation' (Brentano 1973a: 79).

According to Brentano, presentations are the basic units of mental functioning; nothing can be desired or judged until it has first been presented to the mind. Each mental act contains the same object as the presentation to which it is connected: for example, 'nothing is an object of judgement which is not an object of presentation' (Brentano 1973a:

201). There is, he claims, no change in the object towards which we direct the activity of loving, hating, affirming or denying. The nature of the mental act may differ, but the intentional object is unchanged. He claims also that every mental phenomenon is accompanied by the subject's awareness that he is involved in a cognitive process—this is what he calls the 'secondary object'. In the spirit of Descartes' *cogito*, then, it may be possible to question the truth of falsity of an object of thought, but I cannot doubt the fact that I am thinking.

In formulating his account of '*Vorstellung*', Brentano holds the belief that there are two forms of perception. The first is 'external perception'—that is, a sensory perception of a physical phenomenon, such as seeing a colour or hearing a sound. 'Inner perception' (*Innere Wahrnemung*), on the other hand, is a form of reflection on our own ideas. As Linda McAlister puts it: 'mental phenomena are the objects of inner perception, ie. they are what we are conscious of when we introspect' (McAlister 1976: 155).

Freud discusses the notion of *Innere Wahrnemung* in *The Interpretation of Dreams*,[4] stressing that dreams allow better access to unconscious ideas than do waking thoughts:

> In waking life the suppressed material in the mind is prevented from finding expression and is cut off from internal perception ['*Innere Wahrnemung*'] ... (Freud 1900: 608)

Freud's use of the term seems to be consistent with Brentano's notion.[5] At the time, it was unusual to differentiate between 'inner perception' and the received notion of 'introspection'—that is, the attempt to observe your own ideas whilst they occur. Introspection is problematic if you attempt to see yourself seeing yourself, seeing yourself, and so on... *ad infinitum*. However, Brentano avoided this difficulty by claiming that in inner perception one sees what one has just *seen*. In other words, inner perception is a *reflective* process. In order to observe our own ideas or emotions we must wait until they have passed. Brentano provides this example:

> If someone is in a state in which he wants to observe his own anger raging within him, the anger must already be somewhat diminished and so his original object of observation would have disappeared. (Brentano 1973a: 30)

By moving the emphasis from direct observation to *retrospection* Brentano had, he believed, overcome the dilemmas involved in other notions of introspection.

At this point, I would like tot narrow the focus a little in order to emphasise further the extent to which Freud's ideas are in line with Brentano's theory. Brentano's intentionality thesis enables us to differentiate between objects of external perception which are always sensible qualities, and objects of inner perception, which may be *realia* ('things') or *irrealia* ('non-things', such as 'concepts'). According to him, a mental act may be directed towards any object, either physical or imaginary, or towards any other mental act which is not identical with itself.

Brentano taught that every mental act contains an object, although that object need not exist in the extra-mental world. Therefore, the status of a mental object must be considered in a different way from that of a physical entity. While we can be certain that we have had an idea, emotion, etc., we cannot be certain of the truth or falsity of our perceptions of the external world. Linda McAlister puts it this way:

> According to [him], an inner perception is a judgement; it is not an ordinary fallible judgement, however, but rather an evident, ie. self-evidently true, judgement. And all judgements, according to Brentano at that time, were existential in nature, that is to say, they were all either affirmations or denials of the existence of their objects. In the particular case of inner perception, the affirmation of the existence of the object, the mental phenomenon, in question was held by Brentano to be self-evidently true, and so, from the fact that it is the object of this sort of intentional fact, one can infer that the object exists. (McAlister 1976: 157)

However, our sensory perceptions of extended things are deceptive. It is impossible to be certain that our senses reveal the true nature of the sensible world. Physical phenomena merely provide 'signs of something real' (Brentano 1973a: 19). They give an illusion of certainty which may easily be mistaken for 'reality'. He asserts: 'We have no right, therefore, to believe that the objects of so-called external perception really exist as they appear to us. Indeed, they demonstrably do not exist outside of us. In contrast to that which really and truly exists, they are mere phenomena' (Brentano 1973a: 10).

McAlister points out that there is a difference between 'reality' and 'existence' in Brentano's work. For Brentano the expression *'eine Realität'* does not mean the same as something that belongs to the external world. She writes:

> Brentano talks about realia and irrealia (*Realitäten* and *Nichtrealitäten*), about what exists and what does not exist, and he means something different in each case. For Brentano, a realia or *Realität* is a particular individual thing, while an irrealia is a non-thing, as, for example, a universal, a species, a genus, or a state of affairs or values. Brentano maintained that something could be a *Realität*, ie. an individual, a thing, even if it did not exist. A unicorn or hippogriff, for example, would be particular individual things, and hence realia, even though they do not exist. (McAlister 1976: 154)

The same distinction is articulated by Freud. In his 'A Project for a Scientific Psychology' he began to formulate the theory he would later call 'reality-testing'. He explained that an essential function of the ego was its ability to defend itself from the prospect of total belief in hallucinatory fulfilment. There would, for example, be disastrous consequences if one continuously mistook dreams of eating and drinking for reality (Freud 1950: 322-327). This general theme is developed later in Freud's paper of 1925, 'Negation', in which he questions the extent to which we can accept the 'real existence of something of which there is a presentation' (Freud 1925c: 237). He implicitly recognises the difference between external perception and presentations; the latter are *judgements* related to *inner perception*. He has already noted the affirmative judgement of a presentation, in conformity with the pleasure principle, but goes on to explain that:

> The other sort of decision made by the function of judgement—as to the real existence of something of which there is a presentation (reality-testing)—is a concern of the definitive reality ego, which develops out of the pleasure-ego. It is now no longer a question of whether what has been perceived (a thing) shall be taken into the ego or not, but a question of whether something which is in the ego as a presentation can be rediscovered in perception (reality) as well. It is, we see, once more a question of external and internal. What is unreal, merely a presentation and

> subjective, is only internal; what is real is also there outside. (Freud 1925c: 237)

Freud's distinction reflects that made by Brentano. It is fundamental to Brentano's theory of judgement (*Urteil*) that an object is presented to consciousness and affirmed, or presented to consciousness and denied. Brentano's presentations are epistemologically equivalent to those of Freud, although they are based upon mental acts in general, rather than the pleasure/unpleasure sentiment in particular.

We can also compare the Brentanian category of 'love/hate' (*Gemutsbewegungen*) with Freud's 'pleasure principle', which is responsible for acceptance of objects that are good or pleasurable, and for rejection of what is bad or unpleasurable. For Brentano, too, objects presented to consciousness may be loved or hated, pleasurable or unpleasurable. In his 1872-73 lecture notes he holds that 'love/hate' is the instigator of our mental acts. He even suggests that the original motivating force for our actions may be *'lust'* and *'unlust'* (Brentano 1872-73).

In 'Negation', Freud's position is clear. He associates the judgement of affirmation of the *Vorstellung*—or object of presentation—with the pleasure principle. 'Judgement'—that is, the affirmation or denial of the presentation as primary object—is placed within the domain of the reality principle. He writes:

> The function of judgement is concerned in the main with two sorts of decision. It affirms or disaffirms the possession by a thing of a particular attribute; and it asserts or disputes that a presentation has an existence in reality... [T]he original pleasure-ego wants to introject into itself everything that is good and to eject from itself everything that is bad. (Freud 1925c: 236-237)

According to Brentano, everyone has a natural tendency to assent to their own mental acts, to believe in their own ideas. He tells us that 'inner perceptions' are 'true in themselves. As they appear to be, so they are in reality' (Brentano 1973a: 20).

Through experience we learn to judge which of our ideas have been caused by other mental acts, such as fears or desires, and which were caused by the misleading phenomena of the physical world. In his lecture notes, he explains that:

> [O]riginally we instinctively agree to all mental images; and that eventually our trust becomes more limited in sphere, but develops from the instinctive one to an insightful one. Something similar happens in the realm of memory... (cited in Barclay 1964: 20)

In a similar vein, Freud suggests that 'reality testing' begins with sensations which are experienced as persistent physical needs. A baby's first cry may be an instinctive reaction to somatic stimulation, but the emphasis soon shifts from immediate experience to memory. The infant learns to recall this excitation and his own subsequent actions, both mental and physical. Freud writes:

> The antithesis between subject and object does not exist from the first. It only comes into being from the fact that thinking possesses the capacity to bring before the mind once more something that has once been perceived, by reproducing it as a presentation without the external object still having to be there. (Freud 1925c: 237)

The child not only reflects upon an inner perception or idea which is no longer connected to any physical phenomenon, but also the 'reproduction of a perception as a presentation is not always a faithful one; it may be modified by omissions, or changed by the meaning of various elements' (Freud 1925c: 238).

So reality-testing also has the task of discovering the extent of these distortions. In 'Formulations on the Two Principles of Mental Functioning' (1911) we read that:

> With the introduction of the reality principle one species of thought-activity was split off; it was kept free from reality-testing and remained sub-ordinated to the pleasure principle alone. This activity is *phantasying* which... abandons dependence on real objects. (Freud 1911: 222)

From all of this we can conclude that both student and professor share the conviction that psychology is concerned with the 'reality' of ideas, rather than the existence of physical phenomena.

However, Freud did not always follow Brentano's early teachings. In the 1890s he believed in a direct correlation between ideas and external objects. This can be seen in his seduction theory, which asserted that hysteria was always caused by a real(ly existing) event. Freud's subsequent repudiation of the seduction theory represented a return to the conviction that the reality of a belief does not necessarily correspond to something which actually exists.

Thus, for a time, Freud maintained that the hysteric's statement 'I was seduced by my father' corresponded with a state of affairs which existed in the extra-mental world. By assuming this, he failed to make a distinction between an object of inner perception and an object of external perception. The seduction theory carries with it the implication that—in the relevant respect—our knowledge of the world is identical to our judgements concerning our beliefs and desires. In the words of Michael Frampton: 'Freud at first mistakenly inferred from the reality of the intentional act (believing) to the reality of the object of belief (seduction)' (Frampton 1991: 32).[6]

In 'The Aetiology of Hysteria' (1896*c*) Freud argues that all hysterical symptoms can be traced back through chains of associated memories to 'the field of sexual experience' (Freud 1896c: 199). At this point in its history, Freud considered the work of psychoanalysis to consist in discovering the original physical event which later produced hysteria. He writes:

> I therefore put forward the thesis that at the bottom of every case of hysteria there are one or more occurrences of premature sexual experience, occurrences which belong to the earliest years of childhood but which can be reproduced through the work of psychoanalysis in spite of the intervening decades. (Freud 1896c: 203)

It was only when he questioned the ontological status of the immanent object, and returned to the underlying bases of what he had learned from Brentano, that he shifted the emphasis in psychoanalytic practice from 'reality' to 'fantasy'—that is, from existing object to perceptual object. He moved away from the materialistic approach which relied upon observation of the external world, and returned to an intentional thesis.

In 1924 Freud added a footnote to the passage I have just cited from 'The Aetiology of Hysteria': 'it must be remembered that at the time I wrote it I had not yet freed myself from my overvaluation of reality and my low valuation of fantasy' (Freud 1896*c*: 204n).

He came to realise that although the object of a mental act might be caused by a memory of a physical event, it might also be caused by other mental acts, such as wishes or desires. This allowed him to accept that an idea could be real (insofar was it could be affirmed in judgement), even if it did not correspond to an external event. He did accept the hysteric's claim that the seduction was real—*in Brentano's sense*. That is, he attributed the judgement of reality not to a physical event, but to a mental act. In this sense, Freud is drawing upon Brentano's intentionality thesis in his move away from the seduction theory.

I shall close with a quotation from a letter by Freud to Wilhelm Fliess, written in January 1896. Freud writes:

> I see how, via the detour of medical practice, you are reaching your first ideal of understanding human beings as a physiologist, just as I most secretly nourish the hope of arriving, via these same paths, at my initial goal of philosophy. (Masson 1985: 159)

We might hazard the remark that was the elements of Brentano's philosophy which, unrecognised, awaited Freud at this terminus.

Notes

1 See Freud 1989b.

2 *'Vera philosophia methodus nulla alia nisi scientia naturalis est.'* This was one of twenty-five theses Brentano proposed in his Aula on 15th July 1866, at the University of Wurzberg.

3 In 1875 Freud travelled to England to visit his half-brother, Emanuel Freud. According to Peter Gay, this journey marked a decline in Freud's association with Brentano. Gay cites Freud's admiration for the 'consistent empiricism' of English scientists as a reason for this change. He goes on to relate how, as Freud returned from England, '[g]radually the teachings of Brentano were fading into the background' (Gay 1988: 31). Freud left for Manchester on 20th July, 1875, and returned on September 7th of that year. It is true that two days after his return to Vienna, Freud wrote: 'I am more distrustful than ever of philosophy (Freud 1989b: letter of 9th September, 1875). However, as I have pointed out, this is not a comment on the work of Brentano, whose empirical standpoint was still the object of Freud's admiration.

This subsequent remark made by Gay is also misleading: 'In fact, Freud would have little need of philosophy for some time. Upon his return, he began to concentrate on his work in Carl Claus's laboratory' (Gay 1988: 31). Freud did spend two months in Trieste studying with Claus: March-April and September-October, 1876. However, during the intervening summer Freud once again attended Brentano's lectures. This time the course was entitled 'The Philosophy of Aristotle'. This is confirmed in a short article published by Philip Merlan in 1949, in which the author quotes from the archives of the University of Vienna. 'The results show that Freud was enrolled in the courses given by Brentano: in Freud's third, fourth and fifth semesters (Winter 1874/5, Summer 1875, and Winter 1875/6 respectively), "Readings of

Philosophical Writings"; in addition, his fourth semester (Summer 1875) "Logic"; in his sixth semester (Summer 1876), "The Philosophy of Aristotle"' (Merlan 1949: 451).

It is also interesting to note that Carl Claus, the head of the Zoological Institute, with whom Freud worked, was also regularly in attendance at Brentano's lectures.

[4] Indeed, the notion of *Innere* Wahrnemung is implicit in Freud's famous pronouncement that '[t]he interpretation of dreams is the royal road to knowledge of the unconscious activities of the mind' (Freud 1900: 608).

[5] In an editorial footnote to *Psychology from and Empirical Standpoint,* Oscar Krause agrees: 'The question is, whether there can be a state of consciousness not accompanied by a secondary consciousness. Unconscious determining factors [Freud] are quite compatible with this' (Brentano 1973a: 105).

[6] In this quotation Frampton uses the term 'reality' where Brentano would have used 'existing'.

ON FREUD'S ENCOUNTER WITH BRENTANO

Franz Kaltenbeck

In 1870, the University of Vienna was a breeding-ground for ideas which could change a person's life. Indeed, it was far more than a place for simple teaching and learning. The contingencies which determine scientific progress were compounded by chance encounters. Orthodoxy was in jeopardy. A fundamental change of discourse was unfolding.

It is perhaps more helpful to view the Freud-Brentano relationship as an *encounter*, rather than viewing it in terms of influence or as a debt—even though we have only Freud's account on which to base our interpretation. An 'encounter' might be defined as an event which guards against idealism. Indeed, the encounter between Freud and Brentano was not wholly benign; one cannot avoid noticing the sense of trauma which hovers over Freud's account of the visits he paid to his professor of philosophy.

In this chapter I shall examine the circumstances surrounding these visits, in order to shed some light on the concepts of 'God' and 'the cause'. Brentano tended to fuse these notions together. Freud, on the other hand, would eventually separate them.

Historical background

Thanks to *The Letters of Sigmund Freud to Eduard Silberstein 1871-1881* (Freud 1989b), we know that, during the first three years of his studies, Freud was a committed and prominent student member of Brentano's audience.

His encounter with Brentano was foretokened in his correspondence with Silberstein even prior to his enrolment at the university. These letters provide evidence of Freud's ambivalence towards philosophy, and include his attempts at dissuading his friend from taking up the subject.[1] Freud gives the impression of being more at ease with literature, as is shown by his numerous literary allusions to Cervantes, Goethe, Hebbel, and even to Balzac and Poe.

However the nature of his ambivalence towards philosophy—even though it persisted throughout his entire life—is subject to qualification. Firstly, we must consider Freud's unbridled sense of ambition, which was markedly in evidence throughout his whole career. In a letter to Wilhelm Fliess, dated 1st January 1896, he comments on the nature of his ambition as follows:

> The thought that both of us are occupied with the same kind of work is by far the most enjoyable one I can conceive at present. I see how, via the detour of medical practice, you are reaching your first idea of understanding human beings as a physiologist, just as I most secretly nourish the hope of arriving, via these same paths, at my initial goal of philosophy. For that is what I wanted originally, when it was not yet at all clear to me to what end I was in the world. (Masson 1985: 159)

Almost forty years later, we encounter a striking echo of this remark in Freud's 1935 'Postscript' to *An Autobiographical Study*:

> My interest, after making a lifelong *détour* through the natural sciences, medicine and psychotherapy, returned to the cultural problems which had fascinated me long before, when I was a youth scarcely old enough for thinking. (Freud 1935b: 72)

Here, Freud is alluding to works such as *Totem and Taboo, The Future of an Illusion, Civilization and Its Discontents* and *Moses and Monotheism*. Little is known about the source of his interest in the origin of religion, unless one is prepared to consider that here, in 1935, Freud is recalling something which, sixty years earlier, evidently disturbed him a great deal—*the question of the existence of God.*

Taking the two 'confessions' above, of 1896 and of 1935, one might conclude that Freud was closer to Empedocles than to Goethe—closer to the physician-thinker than to the philosopher of nature. In August 1873, during the time of his final examinations, he began reading Aristotle's *Ethica Nicomachaea* and Helmholtz's *Lectures* (Freud 1989b: 49). However, his relationship with philosophy remained irreverent:

> As if the most useless things in the world were not arranged in the following order: shirt collars, philosophers, and monarchs. (Freud 1989b: 52)

He shared this lack of respect for the insignia of the master with other geniuses of his time, who also sought to challenge Emperor

Franz Josef and Bismarck. It might be argued that, at the time, both these men functioned as symbols of the imaginary father, who is cruelly overvalued yet—at the same time—so fragile. Indeed, historians such as Nikolaus Sombart have highlighted the role of this father-figure in the German disaster.[2]

Despite his jests, however, Freud had also become something of a moral aphorist. This is evident in his instructions to Silberstein, for instance, regarding the paradoxes of ethics—that Man suffers just as much from his virtues as from his vices, if he does not curb them.

The visit

Brentano's presence began to exert an effect upon Freud in his second year at university (1874-1875). Freud attended Brentano's courses on metaphysics and J.S. Mill's *Utilitarianism* for four hours each week. Freud the student glowingly extolled his professor of metaphysics:

> One of the courses—listen and marvel!—deals with the existence of God, and Prof. Brentano, who gives the lectures, is a splendid man, a scholar and philosopher, even though he deems it necessary to support this airy existence of God with his own expositions. (Freud 1989b: 70-71)

At the end of the first semester, Freud and his friend Paneth addressed a letter to Brentano which, unfortunately, is lost. The two students expressed their objections to Brentano's proofs of the existence of God. Even so, under Brentano's influence, Freud at this time was contemplating taking a doctorate in philosophy. A timetable from the summer semester shows that Freud registered for the course on 'Logic' taught by the person he described as a

> believer, a teleologist (!) and a Darwinian and a damned clever fellow, a genius in fact, who is, in many respects, an ideal human being. (Freud 1989b: 95)

On the 15th March, 1875, Freud sent Silberstein an account of his visit—with Paneth—to Brentano. The philosopher refuted their objections, telling them that he was well aware they were both materialists. Brentano then launched into a polemic against Herbart and recommended that the two students read Descartes, but avoid Spinoza. As for Leibniz, Locke, Hume and Kant, Brentano insisted they were required reading. The German idealists—on the other hand—he dismissed as 'swindlers'.

Freud was well aware of his master's proclivity for proselytising, even though he had a horror of 'all forms of pathos, or fanaticism'. In the following passage, Freud writes openly about the dilemma with which Brentano confronted him:

> He demonstrates the existence of God with as little bias and as much precision as another might argue the advantage of the wave over the emission theory. Needless to say, I am only a theist by necessity, and am honest enough to confess my helplessness in the face of his argument; however, I have no intention of surrendering so quickly or completely. Over the next few semesters, I intend to make a thorough study of his philosophy, and meanwhile reserve judgement and the choice between theism and materialism. For the time being, I have ceased to be a materialist and am not yet a theist. (Freud 1989b: 104-105)

In his letter dated 11th April, 1875, Freud raised the question of whether the law of causality required the existence of God, and alluded to Kant's refutation of the proofs of the existence of God. The distinction between the analytic and the synthetic proposition was also preying upon his mind, but what perturbed him most was Brentano's own approach to the question, which turned God into 'a logically necessary scientific hypothesis'. Freud wrote:

> The bad part of it, especially for me, lies in the fact that science of all things seems to demand the existence of God... (Freud 1989b: 111)

Perturbing as it may have been, however, one can see clearly that Freud is not entirely convinced by his forced 'conversion'.[3]

Outline of the lectures on metaphysics

Brentano's *Vom Dasein Gottes ('On the Existence of God')* is divided into two parts. The first part deals with the justification of the subject and the ontological proof[4] in the various forms it has adopted during the course of history—for instance, in the works of St Anselm, Descartes and Leibniz. He goes on to examine criticisms of this argument by Hume, Kant, and himself. He replies to Hume and Kant, who both denied the possibility of finding any proof of the existence of the Supreme Being. In the second part, Brentano sets forward his own version of various other proofs—that is, the teleological proof,[5] the proof of the first engine, a proof which rests on contingency, etc.

Brentano's aim in this work is—in opposition to Kant—to show that ethics is based on the sovereign good. This, Brentano asserts, can be ascertained without resorting to a first cause, even though—in the course of his lectures—he denied the possibility of the representation of the sovereign good. In other words, it must be 'the order of the ends' or 'finality' which forms the basis of ethics.

The critique of the ontological proof

On St Anselm's ontological proof, David Lewis writes that although it has never been conclusively refuted neither has it succeeded in converting the non-believer (Lewis 1983: 10-11). Brentano, for his part, believed that Anselm's argument was based on a paralogism. However, this is not why the argument is of interest to us here. To me it seems that these arguments are highly relevant to the problems of *existence* and of the *real* which Freud addressed in 1895—in the 'A Project for a Scientific Psychology'—and again, in 1925, in his essay 'Negation'.

In these works, Freud corrects Anselm, who—in effect—expanded the concept of the real in order to produce 'existence'. For Anselm, existence is a property which things can be said to possess. Freud, on the other hand, conceived of existence as a concept grafted upon a fundamental uncertainty. He addresses the question of whether the search for the lost object will result in the identity of thought (as in 'A Project for a Scientific Psychology' [1950]). Does the object exist? This amounts to the question whether the object can be found in reality (as in 'Negation' [1925c]).

In St Anselm's view, existence is the product of a conceptual operation: God is the most perfect good, hence it is impossible for one to conceive of a more perfect good than God. The argument also relies upon a rather contrived dichotomy between understanding and reality. As Brentano states, the perfect good of God exists in one's understanding from the moment one conceives of it.[6] Accordingly, this leads to the question of knowledge: does this good exist *only* in one's understanding? Decidedly not! Something so perfect—so perfect that nothing surpasses its degree of perfection—cannot exist only in one's understanding, because something which is present in both the realms of understanding and reality is more perfect than that which exists in one's understanding alone. If this were not the case, then there would be something more perfect than that which is so perfect that nothing surpassing its degree of perfection can be conceived of. But, clearly, this is impossible.

Therefore—the argument concludes—God, by necessity, is not only a figment of one's understanding, but also exists in reality.

Brentano elaborates four versions of this line of reasoning. The one based upon Descartes' version of the ontological proof provides a succinct summary of the general argument:

- It is part of God's nature to be indefinitely perfect.
- What is indefinitely perfect is, by its very nature, necessary.
- What is necessary *is*.
- Therefore, God is.

Amongst the critics of this argument, examined by Brentano, I shall mention briefly only Kant. For Kant, every existential proposition is synthetic: that is, 'to be' is *not* a predicate appended to the subject. The existential proposition ('God exists') does not establish a relation between two concepts ('God', 'existence'), but rather between a concept (which fills the slot of the grammatical subject) and the object—that is, the object itself of experience. Hence, Kant refutes the ontological proof in the following way. To paraphrase Kant: 'When I say "God is" I do not posit a new predicate in order to link it to the concept of God. The sole thing this supreme being in my mind lacks is that it cannot be known *a posteriori*. We could refer to the famous joke: that a possible one hundred thalers is equal in amount to one hundred real thalers. However, my fortune will only increase by means of the real hundred thalers.' Comparing the ontological argument with the situation of a merchant who wants to improve his balance sheet by adding a few zeros, Kant wrote: 'An existence outside the domain of one's experience is a presupposition one cannot justify'.[7]

Brentano, however, is not impressed by this refutation. Partly because the Kantian notion of judgement, which entails the link between a concept and the object is, for him, too similar to St Thomas's *comparatio rei et intellectus*. Above all, however, it is the substitution of the predicate by the outside object which Brentano rejects as a monstrous assertion.

Nevertheless, Brentano himself participates in the deconstruction of the argument of St Anselm and Descartes. In his opinion it is flawed by paralogism, due to the equivocal nature of the reasoning. Brentano takes this as an opportunity to introduce his students—on the basis of Aristotle—to an instructive classification of ambiguities in logic, semantics and syntax. If one does not restrict the meaning of this proposition to a definition, then one risks lapsing into the assertion of a false existence: 'There exists a God, and God is an indefinitely perfect being'.

The connection with Freud

Gaunilo of Marmoutier, a contemporary of St Anselm, opposed his famous apologue of the treasure island to the ontological argument. He suggested we consider the legend of an island lost somewhere in the ocean, which is so rich and fertile that no other island on the map can compare with it. If St Anselm were right, argues Gaunilo, this island would have to exist in reality, for if it were purely a figment of our imagination it could not—therefore—be more precious than all the other islands on the map. Gaunilo argues, then, that z Anselm's argument presupposes what he has to prove—that is, the real being.

The same criticism cannot be levelled at Freud. Take, for instance, the chapter entitled 'Cognition and Reproductive Thought' in the 'Project'. Here Freud is not concerned at all with defining reality *a priori*. Instead, he constructs a mechanism which allows the subject to recognise the desired object as *not being real*. In sum, reality depends upon a process of refutation.

The case in which the mnemic image, invested with desire, co-exists with the perception of this image is of no interest. However, when the desire and the perception tally only partially, it is a different matter. In this case, '[a] way is now found of completing the similarity into an identity' (Freud 1950: 328). Freud describes this path as 'judgement'. As can be seen, reality is introduced only negatively as that which *must not* be mistaken for the object of desire. Furthermore, perfection is a result and not the predicate of a premise. Perfection is an identity which rests upon a judgement—that is, upon an act of thought.

There have been many comments on the two types of judgement which are present in negation: the attributive judgement and the judgement of existence. The latter concerns 'the real existence of something of which there is a presentation' (Freud 1925c: 237). Freud writes:

> It is now no longer a question of whether what has been perceived (a thing) shall be taken into the ego or not, but of whether something which is in the ego as a presentation can be rediscovered in perception (reality) as well. (Freud 1925c: 237)

I shall emphasise two points in this passage. Firstly, Freud's judgement of existence shares with Kant the fact that one of the terms is present in reality—that is, it is an object. The second term, for Kant, is a *concept*; for Freud, it is a *representation*. However, Freud's conception differs radically from Kant's with the introduction of the verb 'to recover' in his notion of judgement. This indicates that, for Freud, an action is involved, and not a simple relation along the lines of a *comparatio*—as Brentano described it in his criticism of Kant. It becomes apparent, then, that the product of this judgement (truth) is incumbent upon the subject. In my opinion, in his critique of judgement, Deleuze overlooked this dynamic aspect in the Freudian judgement of existence.[8]

My second point concerns the auxiliary verb which transforms the Freudian judgement of existence into a modal statement: 'whether something... *can* be rediscovered'. This modal auxiliary puts the Freudian judgement of existence on the spot: the result of the judgement, indeed, might go either way. It is this modality which aims at the notion of cause.

The lack of evidence for the existence of God

The existence of God is by no means self-evident. According to Brentano, only inner perception is able to provide us with 'immediate and unambiguous evidence' (Brentano 1973b: 128-129). Before writing the 'Project', Freud was inspired by the philosopher Wilhelm Jerusalem's *Die Urteilsfunction* (1895). Jerusalem, like Freud and—subsequently—Wittgenstein, contested the evidence of inner perception.[9]

Descartes was wrong: we cannot claim to possess an adequate idea or representation of God. It would be pointless to infer the cause from such an idea. But if there is no evidence to substantiate this, or if the ontological argument is considered invalid, one might look for other proofs. Brentano proposes four options, which he elaborates on a scientific basis, apparently in the hope of rendering them more credible. His allusions to Darwinism, the theory of probability, the paradoxes of the infinite, and to thermodynamics, add a scientific dimension to his philosophical erudition. This stimulated the young Freud, who was later to engage with some of the figures mentioned in these lectures: Helmholtz, Darwin, Weismann, Fechner, and Du Bois-Reymond. In the course of these lectures Freud was introduced to the philosophies of Heraclitus and Empedocles, which would later resonate throughout *Beyond the Pleasure Principle*.

Evidently, then, Brentano sought to replace the 'concept' with 'cause'.

- There is nothing in the realm of our experience which is of immediate necessity.
- Instead, immediate necessity is transcendental.
- Furthermore, it is a creative principle which:
    1) is capable of *ex nihilo* creation
    2) needs no subject to record its effects
- In contrast to Aristotle, Brentano does not conceive of immediate necessity as devoid of change.
- Finally, the immediate necessity, for Brentano, is an *understanding*.

Brentano supports his argument in the following fashion. If the first principle—which creates *ex nihilo*—were to operate blindly, it would be multiple instead of one. Indeed, a uniform principle would only be able to create uniformity. This is in contradiction with the fact that the world is multiple. Therefore, the argument continues, there must be several first principles. Furthermore, these first principles must have various dimensions, such as space. Understanding lacks extention. Therefore, the first principle must be an understanding. And since it is not devoid of change, it must have its proper mode of change—that is, knowledge of the past and future.

Overdetermination

I will mention two points which follow on from this line of reasoning, both of which have a bearing on Freud's ideas.

The first concerns Freud's earliest constructions of the psychical apparatus. These evolve in space: as a framework in the 'Project', as a system of re-transcription in Letter 112 (Masson 1985: 207-15), and—

finally—the optical model used in *The Interpretation of Dreams.* Understanding, here, is the objective and not the cause of these constructions.

Secondly, Freud does not reduce the multiple to the one. Within the Freudian elaboration of causality, multiple causes are referred to as the 'overdetermination' of the symptom or of the dream. Freud touched upon the dialectics of the multiple and the one in 1939 and—exactly as stated by Brentano—he considers it biased in favour of the one. In *Moses and Monotheism* Freud asserts:

> These are perfectly justifiable lines of approach [concerning the impact of individuals on the course of history], but they give us occasion for drawing attention to an important discrepancy between the attitude taken up by our organ of thought and the arrangement of things in the world, which are supposed to be grasped by means of our thought. It is enough for our need to discover causes (which, to be sure, is imperative) if each event has *one* demonstrable cause. But in the reality lying outside us that is scarcely the case; on the contrary, each event seems to be overdetermined and proves to be the effect of several convergent causes. (Freud 1939: 107)

The same applies to the idea of monotheism. It is not the property of Moses. He defended this idea, but this activity is situated in a chain of causes which passes from his predecessor—Akhenaten—and continues through the prophets.

Freud reserves 'a place for the "great man" in the chain, or rather the network, of causes' (Freud 1939: 108). The 'great man' is the father. The father's image, however, is a complex of characteristics—the 'traits of the father': decisiveness, force of will, power of action, independence.

By deconstructing both God and the father Freud corrected an error committed by Brentano who—in Lacan's words—had left the 'weight of the cause on God's shoulders' (Lacan 1984).

Notes

1 See Freud 1989b: 52. Letter dated 22nd August, 1874.

2 See Sombart 1987.

[3] The lectures on Logic given by Brentano between 1874 and 1895 are collected in Brentano 1956, whilst the lectures on metaphysics have been published as Brentano 1980.

[4] [The ontological argument is an *a priori* argument for the existence of God. It is founded on the assumption that existence is a property. Since God is perfect, this property must be an attribute of God by His very nature, otherwise He would fall short of perfection if He existed only in the mind, instead of in the mind *and* in reality. Thus God, by His very nature, necessarily possesses existence.—*Ed.*]

[5] [The teleological argument is the *a posteriori* argument for the existence of God based on the assumption that order in the universe implies an orderer, and thus cannot be an accidental feature of the universe.—*Ed.*]

[6] Brentano formulates this premise in exactly the same way as Daniel Paul Schreber.

[7] Kant deals at length with the ontological proof in his *Critique of Pure Reason* (Kant 1986: 500-7).

[8] See Deleuze's commentary on judgement (Deleuze 1993: 158-169).

[9] See Kaltenbeck 1985.

JOHN STUART MILL TRANSLATED BY SIGMUND FREUD

Michael Molnar

Introduction

Because this chapter is concerned with influences and associations of ideas, and because this is notoriously imprecise territory, I want to start begin with a specific date: 6 May, 1856. This date has a peculiar significance for Freud's pre-analytic work; it was the day on which the famous Scottish philosopher Sir William Hamilton died.

There are only two books by J.S. Mill in Freud's library in London. One is the volume of Freud's translations of Mill undertaken for Theodor Gomperz, the editor of Mill's works in German. I shall return to that later. The other is Mill's *An Examination of Sir William Hamilton's Philosophy*. Now, although Freud did not literally translate this book, in a metaphorical sense certain ideas found in it were to be 'translated' into Freud's idiom.

Mill's book on Hamilton was published in 1865, but Freud's copy is the sixth edition, published in 1889. Freud used it as part of his background reading for *On Aphasia*, where he cites it, together with Mill's *System of Logic*, in part VI, referring especially to the chapter 'Of the Things denoted by Names' in Mill's *System of Logic* (Freud 1992: 122). In the aphasia study Freud is at that point discussing the idea that the word acquires meaning by being linked to an object-presentation, and this object-presentation borrows its verisimilitude only from an assumed chain of associations. These ideas of object- and word- presentation, first presented in *On Aphasia*, are to recur in 'The Unconscious' as the traits differentiating conscious from unconscious mental activity. Hence this philosophical (or linguistic) notion is of vital significance.

What we see here is an interaction between language and consciousness which impinges on one of the nineteenth century philosophical debates that Mill examines in his book on Hamilton—for example, in his discussion of the dispute between Nominalists (who denied general substance and held there was nothing general except names) and Conceptualists (who held that generality is an attribute not only of names but of thoughts). Mill placed Hamilton among the conceptualists. In chapter XVII of his Hamilton study—'The Doctrine of

Concepts, or General Notions'—Mill depicts Hamilton's version of naming as founded on concepts which are in effect a set of unconscious relationships. According to Hamilton 'a concept cannot, as such, be 'realised in thought', or 'elicited into consciousness'' (Mill 1889: 402). There is an intriguing overlap here between this philosophical debate and the schema of an unconscious structured like a language. To follow that parallel would take me beyond the scope of this chapter, so I can only indicate here this nineteenth century area of discussion, in which the hypothesis of unconscious mental activity was being subjected to philosophical and linguistic scrutiny.[1]

Associationism versus Intuitionism

I am not going to argue that the source of the psychoanalytical unconscious can be unearthed in a now rather obscure philosophical polemic between Mill and Hamilton. But Mill's book on Hamilton, if not a direct cause of any specific subsequent development in Freud, at the very least gave him a ringside seat at some of the seminal intellectual debates of that era. Apart from the linguistic question I have mentioned, we also encounter here the philosophico-psychological debate, between intuitionism and associationism. John Stuart Mill, and his father James Mill before him, were committed to the theory that the mind functions and perceives the world through a system of mental associations. Sir William Hamilton was the most eminent representative of the antagonistic philosophy that argued in favour of intuitive knowledge.

There are two things to note here. One is that up to this time there is not always a clear distinction between philosophy and psychology. Much of Locke, Hume or Berkeley could be classified as psychological speculation. Though psychology emerges as a scientific field in the nineteenth century it is still looking towards philosophy for corroboration, and philosophers were still involved in problems now consigned to psychology.[2] The second point about Mill's polemic with Hamilton, and one that gives it resonance, is that the quarrel between associationists and intuitionists had wide-reaching social, religious and political repercussions. In his *Autobiography* Mill wrote:

> The notion that truths external to the mind may be known by intuition or consciousness, independently of observation and experience, is, I am persuaded, in these times, the great intellec-

> tual support of false doctrines and bad institutions. By the aid of this theory, every inveterate belief and every intense feeling, of which the origin is not remembered, is enabled to dispense with the obligation of justifying itself by reason, and is erected into its own all sufficient voucher and justification. There never was such an instrument devised for consecrating all deep seated prejudices. (Mill 1971: 134)

Thus Mill's confrontation with Hamilton's philosophy is an important battle in the long-running war between liberal politics and political reaction, or between the rule of reason and the rule of faith.[3]

The principle of the association of ideas had already been adopted by David Hartley as the basis for a psychology in the eighteenth century: it was to be taken over by Jeremy Bentham as the foundation of the deterministic psychology underpinning his utilitarianism. Through Bentham the idea is passed down to James Mill and to his son John Stuart Mill.[4]

Now all these writers were on Freud's reading list in the 1870s. In his letter to Eduard Silberstein of 22nd/23rd October, 1874, Freud mentions Brentano's lectures on Mill's *Utilitarianism.* In the letter of 15th March, 1875 he writes that Brentano recommends his pupils to study Locke and Hume, and also that he spoke of Hume as the most exemplary of the philosophers (Freud 1989a). Brentano had just published his *Psychologie vom empirischen Standpunkt* in 1874, in which, among other things, he examined the psychology of Hamilton and the Mills. In 1875, then, when Freud was following Brentano's psychology course, they were discussing both Mill and the 'Laws of Association of Ideas'. In short, without having to prove that Freud read every word of the writings of Hume, Locke, Bentham, the Mills etc., one can assume that he was aware of the outlines of this particular associationist tradition.

But how does this 'cultural translation' relate to Freud's literal translation of four essays by Mill? There is a wider- and a narrower-scale answer to that. On the wider scale, J.S. Mill was for the mid-nineteenth century a *Kulturträger*, a figure who embodied a liberal political, social and philosophical tradition. Now although Freud did the translations for Gomperz as a piece of hackwork, for the money, we cannot ignore the fact that Mill commanded the respect of anyone fighting for progress at this time. What persuaded and motivated Freud to undertake the job was probably not the money alone, but also respect for the author—and for his editor Gomperz, who had become a German representative of that tradition. This incentive may well have been reinforced by Freud's strong desire for self-improvement—the 1870s were his most autodidactic phase.

On the narrower scale, what relevance did the Mill essays have to Freud's interests at the time, or to the linguistic and associationist traditions I have mentioned? Only one of the essays is specifically about philosophy, more exactly about Plato. At first sight even this appears remote from Freud's reading at that time or the philosophical battle between associationism and intuitionism that was so important for Mill. But Mill never forgets that Plato is a sounding board for contemporary problems, and on closer reading we can find echoes of the associationist controversy. An example of this is Mill's discussion of the platonic distinction between 'opinion' and 'knowledge', in which Mill decidedly co-opts Plato for his own empirical, rationalist cause[5]:

> True Opinion is converted into knowledge, when bound down… "by a chain of causal reasoning"… This binding process, it is added, is… reminding, and can only be accomplished by questioning, sufficiently repeated and diversified. (Mill 1979: vol. XI, 430)

Freud would have been fully aware of the polemic background when he very faithfully translated such passages. He would have certainly had to consider carefully how to render such terms as 'a chain of causal reasoning' ('*eine Kette ursächlichen Raisonnements*' [Mill 1880: 97]).

Laborious Translation

This preamble finally brings me, via that 'chain of causal reasoning', to the issue of the translation as a translation. What first induced me to look at the Mill translation, simply in terms of its accuracy, was a statement in Jones' biography:

> In the first part of the year [1879] Freud was able to cope with the boredom [of military service] by devoting himself to translating a book by John Stuart Mill, the first of five large books he translated. It was congenial work, since he was specially gifted as a translator. Instead of laboriously transcribing from the foreign

> language, idioms and all, he would read a passage, close the book and consider how a German writer would have clothed the same thoughts—a method not very common among translators. (Jones 1953, p. 61)

As a translator myself, I was highly intrigued by this, and imagined Sigmund Freud reading a page, closing the book, then working from memory into the German translation. If he had used this method, his German version would obviously reveal different turns of phrase, idioms, and in general a new perspective that could very likely provide insight into his reading of Mill's work. Consequently, on comparison of the two texts, I must admit I was disappointed to find how exact and faithful Freud's version actually is. In fact it is as near word for word as possible. It is as if, given the constraints of differing syntax, Freud had indeed 'laboriously transcribed' from the foreign language. This casts some doubt on Jones's assertion. Taken together with his implication that other translators usually 'transcribe' the idioms of the source language into the target language—a statement which betrays total ignorance of translation in general—I can only conclude that his comment on Freud's translation is (to put it mildly) misleading.

One possible motive for Jones's version is that he wished to provide evidence for Freud's extraordinary memory. But even if Freud retained his photographic memory up to 1879, what would be the point of using it while translating, if he was simply arriving at a version identical to that which would have resulted from keeping the original in front of him? The only conceivable purpose would be showing off—but to whom?—or jumping through hoops for the sake of it. Furthermore, any outside evidence for Jones' account is lacking. I can only assume that it arose from some misinterpretation of Freud's comment on his work technique. After all, how long is a 'passage': a long sentence? A paragraph? And as for looking up from the original while thinking of the translation, this is no more than standard practice.

At any rate, there are very few deviations from Mill's text, even in terms of sentence structure, subordinate clauses etc. The changes, where they occur, are subtle. I will present one example, chosen simply because it is about the art of translation:

> We lose, of course, Plato's dramatic power, his refined comedy, and the magic of his style, the reproduction of which (could any one hope to succeed in it) would be the work, not of an exposi-

> tor, but of a translator. But the thoughts are there, exactly as they are, and exactly where they are, in the Platonic writings. (Mill 1979: 383)

> Zwar geht uns Plato's dramatische Gewalt, seine feine Ironie und der Zauber seines Styls verloren, dessen Wiedergabe—wenn man überhaupt hoffen könnte, dieß zu erreichen—die Aufgabe eines Übersetzers, nicht eines Erklärers wäre; aber alle Gedanken Plato's finden wir wieder genau wie und genau wo sie in den platonischen Schriften erscheinen. (Mill 1880: 38-39)

It is interesting that Freud translates 'refined comedy' as *'feine Ironie'*—which, in Mill's terms, is an act of exposition rather than translation. Apart from that, the only other noticeable change here is that Freud has made two sentences out of one. Mill's sentence 'But the thoughts are there...' has been turned into a clause following a semicolon. This is something Freud has done in other places too. It is as if his translation is trying to stress the flow of thought. However, it does this at the expense of conciseness. In a way, this is paradoxical. Mill was no stylist, and his writing is often ponderous and convoluted. In a letter of 15th November, 1883 to Martha Bernays, Freud complained of the lifeless style of these essays—'Ich schimpfte damals über seinen leblosen Stil'—and of the lack of wit and aphorisms (Freud 1960b: 81). Lengthening his sentences would tend, if anything, to exaggerate that fault, and I am tempted to ascribe that to the translator's irritation with the original, but do not consider this one piece of ambiguous evidence on its own as adequate proof.[6]

The Forced Subordination of Women

This leads to questions of style and sympathy. In a study of Freud's translation in terms of its professional standard, Margareta Bowen states that one of the tests of a good translator is the ability to provide accurate translations even where the translator is not in sympathy with the form or content of the original.[7] On the evidence of the Taylor essay, and knowing Freud's complaints to his fiancée about this work, Bowen concludes that Freud passes this test. I agree that he does, but not quite with an *A+*. A mistranslation has crept in at one point in the following passage:

> It requires unusual moral courage as well as disinterestedness in a woman, to express opinions favourable to women's enfranchisement, until, at least, there is some prospect of obtaining it. The comfort of her individual life and her social consideration, usually depend on the good-will of those who hold undue power, and to possessors of power any complaint, however bitter, of the misuse of it, is a less flagrant act of insubordination than to protest against the power itself. The professions of women in this matter remind us of the State offenders of old, who, on the point of execution, used to protest their love and devotion to the sovereign by whose unjust mandate they suffered. (Mill 1979: 40)

The deviant sentence from Freud's German translation reads:

> ...und Machthabern erscheint keine noch so bittere Klage über den Mißbrauch ihrer Gewalt als ein ebenso schreiender Act der Widersetzlichkeit wie eine Anfechtung dieser Macht selbst. (Mill 1880: 27)

What Freud has done here is to turn 'a less flagrant act' into its negative, 'a *no less* flagrant act'. The effect of this is to negate the sense of Harriet Taylor's argument. She is saying that those in power can put up even with bitter complaints against the abuse of power, so long as the complainer does not attack the source of power itself. Freud has made her say the opposite—that those in power see *any* complaint as an attack on the source of power itself. The effect is to undermine an important point about the situation of women; they are permitted to complain about anything except the true source of all their complaints. By exaggerating female limitations and male tyranny, Freud's version caricatures the woman's point of view and ignores woman's actual perspective.

As a translator myself, and therefore inhabitant of a glass house, I would be inclined to invoke Timpanaro's naturalistic reading of parapraxes against Freud's own psychopathology, and say that lack of attention, without unconscious intent, could easily have caused such a slip. However, one already knows Freud's lack of sympathy for women's rights, which makes the plea of extenuating circumstances difficult in this instance. The attack on the essay, in Freud's letter of 15th November, 1883 to Martha Bernays, must be taken seriously as a political statement, for it is reinforced by the fact that Freud was to make similar remarks twenty-five years later, to the Vienna Psychoanalytic Society on March 11, 1908.

The presentation was by Wittels on 'The Natural Position of Women'. In the discussion Freud said:

> In an essay on woman's bondage, John Stuart Mill has overlooked the fact that a woman cannot earn a living and raise children at the same time. Women as a group profit nothing by the modern feminist movement; at best a few individuals profit. (Nunberg & Federn 1962-75: 351)

But Taylor (and Mill) did not overlook that fact: Freud had forgotten, or chose to forget, statements he himself had once translated:

> It is neither necessary nor just to make imperative on women that they shall be either mothers or nothing; or that if they have been mothers once, they shall be nothing else during the whole remainder of their lives. (Mill & Mill 1983: 17)

> There is no need to make provision by law that a woman shall not carry on the active details of a household, or of the education of children, and at the same time practice a profession, or be elected to parliament. Where incompatibility is real, it will take care of itself: but there is gross injustice in making of incompatibility a pretence for the exclusion of those in whose case it does not exist. (Mill & Mill 1983: 18)

Whether or not the movement for women's enfranchisement had by then achieved much for the common woman was beside the point, which is one of human rights and political justice. As Harriet Taylor said (again, a passage Freud had translated):

> But, in truth, none of these arguments and considerations touch the foundations of the subject. The real question is, whether it is right and expedient that one-half of the human race should pass through life in a state of forced subordination to the other half. (Mill & Mill: 23)

It cannot even be argued that Freud was typical of his time as far as his views on the position of women was concerned, at least not if we are speaking of liberal public opinion. When the 1867 Reform Act was being discussed by the British Parliament, J.S. Mill proposed giving women the vote. (Part of the discussion hinged on a linguistic question. Mill sardonically turned patriarchal terminology against itself, arguing that in law the term 'man' subsumed that of 'woman' and therefore a vote for manhood suffrage automatically included female suffrage.) The proposal was defeated, predictably but not overwhelmingly. 196 voted against, 73 voted in favour.[8] Judging Freud, therefore, not by the puristic standards of late twentieth century political correctness, but by those of his time, he was—in this respect—a reactionary. It is as if, in the case of women's political rights, Freud has done exactly what Jones said he did when he translated; he read Mill and then closed the book.

Free Association: Macaulay and Milton

Though Freud rejected Harriet Taylor's political message, in view of his social-democratic tendencies he probably read the essay on socialism with more sympathy.[9] Also he may well have learnt something of Greek philosophy from the Plato essay. (The only work of Plato remaining in his library is the Symposium.) But, as far as style rather than content is concerned, Freud fortunately learnt nothing from these essays. He had already started to develop what a teacher had praised as his 'idiotic' style, and he had enough aesthetic sense not to let it be influenced by philosophical jargon. At the same time he was a good enough translator not to impose his own style on Mill. Consequently these four essays are, stylistically, a foreign body in Freud's work—they do not sound at all like the Freud we know.

That is not to say that they do not form part of his intellectual idiom, for the questions they debate belong firmly to the culture that formed him. Among those formative influences are the traditions of British empirical philosophy and psychology which Mill mediated. But there are some other corollaries of British culture—and ones that Freud might have seen as a sort of antidote to Mill—which ought to be invoked somewhere on the margins, or here at the end of this study of influences and associations.

In the letter to Silberstein of 10th August, 1879 in which Freud reports working on Mill's Plato, he speaks with great enthusiasm of reading two volumes of Macaulay's essays.[10] On 24th September, 1879, a month after finishing the Mill translation (and perhaps even with the money he received for it?) Freud acquired a two-volume edition of Milton's poetry. Now Macaulay and Milton are two of the notable writers Freud mentioned in his response to Hugo Heller's questionnaire on 1st November, 1906, and the two come together in Macaulay's essay on Milton. A passage from that essay may serve here as a sort of summary of some of the philosophical, psychological and linguistic themes I have mentioned:

> The most striking characteristic of the poetry of Milton is the extreme remoteness of the associations by means of which it acts on the reader. Its effect is produced, not so much by what it expresses, as by what it suggests; not so much by the ideas which it directly conveys, as by other ideas which are connected with them. He electrifies the mind through conductors. (Macaulay 1924: 157).

Macaulay continues this passage, in a similarly highly charged vein, speaking of the power of names and naming in Milton's poetry. I should like this quotation to be read not only as an oblique comment on the mode of connection between Freud's early work and the later, canonised Freud, but also as a reference back to the philosophical and psychological debates on language and naming with which I began:

> Every one of them [the names] is the first link in a long chain of associated ideas. Like the dwelling place of our infancy revisited in manhood, like the song of our country heard in a strange land, they produce upon us an effect wholly independent of their intrinsic value. (Macaulay 1924: 158)

Notes

[1] In *An Autobiographical Study* Freud refers contemptuously to 'the philosophers, for whom 'conscious' and 'mental' were identical, and who protested that they could not conceive of such an absurdity as the 'unconscious mental'' (Freud 1925b: 31). But who are these unnamed, ridiculed philosophers? Certainly not Schopenhauer or Nietzsche. Brentano is the first likely candidate, but second in line is J.S. Mill. In *An Examination of Sir William Hamilton's Philosophy*, and particularly in Chapter XV ('Sir William Hamilton's Doctrine of Unconscious Mental Modifications'), Mill argues against certain unconscious states of mind posited by

Hamilton, among them unconscious mental associations. For Mill these are the trappings of intuitionism, with all its concomitant social and political evils.

[2] Alan Ryan in his introduction to Mill's *Examination of Sir William Hamilton's Philosophy* states: 'The argument between Mill and Hamilton is, in their terms, an argument about the nature and contents of 'consciousness'; it is in some sense an argument about psychological issues' (Mill 1979). And among Mill's many concerns is one that affected Freud too, namely the debate on the connections of science and philosophy. At the opening of his book on Hamilton, Mill stresses that fields of enquiry overlap and that 'the difficulties of Metaphysics lie at the root of all science' (Mill 1889: 2).

[3] The philosophical history of this particular conflict goes back at least to Locke. In *An Essay Concerning Human Understanding* (1689) we find Locke arguing against the doctrine of innate propositions, a notion that was used as the basis of the view that there were certain principles that could not be questioned. Locke's antidote to the rule of faith was a rationally grounded explanation of understanding and behaviour. Fifty years after Locke, in his *Treatise of Human Nature*, Hume was asserting that causation itself is based on an association of ideas, that is, on human perception: 'We have no other notion of cause and effect, but that of certain objects, which have been *always conjoined* together' (Hume 1970: 140). This philosophy requires, and is ratified by, psychology. Both Locke and Hume were straddling fences; for us their empirical approach seems to confuses philosophical theory and psychological hypothesis.

[4] According to Bertrand Russell (who was, incidentally, J.S. Mill's god-son): 'To Bentham, determinism in psychology was important, because he wished to establish a code of laws—and, more generally, a social system—which would automatically make men virtuous' (Russell 1961: 741).

As far as J.S. Mill and Bentham are concerned, Andrew Watson has traced a line of contact between them and Freud. He draws comparisons between Freud's pleasure principle and Bentham's utilitarian philosophy, quoting Bentham's *An Introduction to the Principles of Morals and Legislation* (1789), which opens with the statement: 'Nature has placed mankind under the governance of two sovereign masters, *pain and pleasure*. It is for them alone to point out what we ought to do, as well as determine what we shall do. On the one hand the standard of right and wrong, on the other the chain of cause and effect, are fastened to their throne.' (Watson 1958: 326).

[5] Though the German translation of this essay is simply entitled *Plato*, in English it was *Grote's Plato*: an extended review and discussion of Grote's edition of Plato. In preparation for the review Mill reread the entire works of Plato in Greek and the review presents a Plato in his own image, based upon the order of production of Plato's works established by Grote: 'He [Plato] probably became indifferent to speculation for its own sake, ceased to expect that any theoretical position would be found unassailable, and no longer cared for anything but practical results.' (Mill 1979: 431). Grote's order of production has, however, since been modified, so that this quasi-utilitarian image of Plato is no longer viable (Mill 1979: xxxix-xl).

[6] It should not be forgotten that one of the essays, *The Enfranchisement of Women*, was actually written by Mill's wife, Harriet Taylor, a fact Mill stresses in his publication of the text and which Gomperz briefly acknowledges in a footnote. As Mill's publication of the essay was an act of love and submission to Harriet Taylor, so Gomperz's edition was an expression of laborious devotion to Mill, a devotion that had at one time manifested itself as passionate and unrequited love for Mill's step-daughter Helen Taylor, who turned him down, and was to refuse any marriage, in order to take care of her widowed step-father. The shattering of his delusional love precipitated a brief psychotic episode in Gomperz. In his edition of his father's letters (a work Freud possessed in his library), Heinrich Gomperz stated: 'man kann sich des Eindrucks kaum erwehren, was Th. G. beglückte, sei weniger die Aussicht gewesen, Helen Taylors Gatte, als vielmehr die, Mills Schwiegersohn zu werden' (Gomperz 1936: 322).

Harriet Taylor's essay, in highlighting key issues of the relationship of the sexes, goaded Freud into a refutation of Taylor and Mill's position at the Vienna Psychoanalytic Society as late as 1908, and in a letter to his fiancée of 15th November, 1883 he is arguing against Mill and Taylor in his attempt to justify his patriarchal attitude towards Martha. In this connection it is worth noting a couple of small but indicative disparities in Freud's translation. Firstly the title—*Ueber Frauenemancipation*—is slightly inaccurate: emancipation is liberation in general, whereas enfranchisement is a more precise concept, namely attainment of the right to vote. Secondly, a very subtle alteration occurs in Taylor's passage on the ideal of marriage. She says: 'The highest order of durable and happy attachments would be a hundred times more frequent than they are, if the affection which the two sexes sought from one another were that genuine friendship, which only exists between equals in privileges as in faculties' (Mill & Mill 1983: 34). Here Freud has translated the last words as 'between equals in privileges and faculties' ('die einander an Rechten und an Fähigkeiten gleich sind' [Mill 1880: 23]). By translating 'as in' as 'and' Freud glosses over a contrast Taylor implies, between faculties that are already equal and privileges that are still lacking.

[7] My thanks to Lydia Marinelli for supplying me with a copy of this article.

[8] In his *Autobiography*, Mill described this as 'perhaps the only really important public service I performed in the capacity of a Member of Parliament: a motion to strike out the words which were understood to limit the electoral franchise to males, thereby admitting to the suffrage all women who as householders or otherwise possess the qualification required of male electors… But it was as yet uncertain whether the proposal would obtain more than a few stray votes in the House: and when, after a debate in which the speakers on the contrary side were conspicuous by their feebleness, the votes record in favour of the motion amounted to 73—made up by pairs and tellers to above 80—the surprise was general and the encouragement great...' (Mill 1971: 179).

[9] Such passages as the following might have caught Freud's attention (and have still not lost their immediacy): 'The one certainty is that Communism, to be successful, requires a high standard of moral and intellectual education in all members of the community...' (Mill 1879: 522). 'But to force unprepared populations into Communist societies, even if a political revolution gave the power to make such an attempt, would end in disappointment' (Mill 1879: 523).

[10] Two years earlier, in the Silberstein letter of 7th September, 1877, Freud had already expressed his delight at Macaulay's essays, especially praising the ones on William Temple and Francis Bacon. It is worth noting here that, when Freud started publicly doubting the authorship of Shakespeare, there was never a whisper of Bacon's name, although his claim is no less feasible than that of Freud's candidate, the Earl of Oxford. If we want to find a reason we need go no further than this essay of Macaulay's, which is a thorough character assassination of Bacon. Having read it, no one could believe the petty-minded, treacherous little man that Macaulay portrays might be remotely capable of writing Shakespeare's plays.

FREUD, HYSTERIA, AND PSYCHIATRY AS THE IMPOSSIBLE PROFESSION

Aisling Campbell

In 'Analysis Terminable and Interminable', Freud speaks of the professions of analysis, government and teaching as the 'impossible professions' (Freud 1937: 248). Psychiatry is a science which, like analysis, is directly concerned with the human subject, but which has moved away from a concern with the *particular* of the subject to become a science of the *general*, of classification and criteria. The result is a master discourse which embodies an impossibility. As such, psychiatry has become the epitome of the impossible profession and its practitioners, not surprisingly, feel pessimistic about its future.

It is hysteria which poses the greatest problem for psychiatry. Given the question of trauma with which psychiatry concerns itself, we must ask 'how can psychiatry address the hysterical subject?' This question implies that psychiatrists must seek to know about the *history* of the subject. In this case it seems appropriate to look to the history of the Freudian relation with hysteria.

Freud's pre-analytic writings are viewed as constitutive of psychoanalysis, but are also axiomatically claimed as part of the history of psychiatry and, indeed, of the plethora of 'behavioural sciences'. However, this history is not a pre-determined, linear progression. It reveals an *oscillation* on Freud's part in terms of his relation to hysteria. This oscillation is repeated in the present-day psychiatric approach to trauma. The kernel of this repetition is *the real*, which is thrown into relief by the inadequacy of the symbolic order and is itself constitutive of trauma. In order to situate the dilemma of modern psychiatry in relation to hysteria I shall examine some of Freud's early writings on the subject.

It is often said that Freud was forced to abandon his mastery of the subject(s) of hysteria in order to achieve a position of ignorance and thus to discover the importance of speech. However, Freud's studies in Paris predated his mastery of hysteria and—it seems to me—in an almost hysterical way Freud sought a master-figure in Charcot as a response to his own questioning of hysteria. In his 'Paris Report' (Freud 1956) Freud protests somewhat too much, we might think, about the poor facilities at the laboratories of the Salpêtrière. He was forced to abandon his neuropathological studies after the discovery of the restiform nucleus.[1] He tells us that:

> Some extremely valuable pathological material was put at my disposal; but I found that the conditions for making use of it were most unfavourable. The laboratory was not at all adapted to the reception of an extraneous worker, and such space and resources as existed were made inaccessible owing to lack of any kind of organisation. (Freud 1956: 8)

We wonder if the lack of organisation may have been partly Freud's! The contrast between Freud's attitude towards the laboratory and the clinic, however, makes his decision to continue his studies under Charcot seem inevitable:

> In contrast to the inadequacy of the laboratory, the clinic at the Saltpêtrière provided such a plethora of new and interesting material that it needed all my efforts to profit by the instruction which this favourable opportunity afforded. (Freud 1956: 9)

Freud was unstinting in his praise of Charcot, yet we may also infer from his commentary that Charcot was diligent in his refusal of this position of master. 'The whole trend of his mind', says Freud, 'leads me to suppose that he can find no rest till he has correctly described and classified some phenomenon with which he is concerned but that he can sleep quite soundly without having arrived at the physiological explanation of that phenomenon' (Freud 1956: 13).

The choice that Freud made between the study of neuroanatomy and the study of hysteria is surely a founding moment in the history of psychoanalysis. This was not due to mere chance—and certainly not only due to the poorly organised laboratories in the Salpêtrière—but was bound up with Freud's own desire.

From 'A Case of Hemi-Anaesthesia in a Hysterical Male' (Freud 1886d) we obtain a sense of Freud's fascination with the origins of the symptoms of the patient. The vividness of his description, which includes even the events leading up to the development of hemianaesthesia, betrays Freud's seduction by this hysteric. Quite apart from the liveliness of the account, it is clear that Freud *listened* to his patient. We are given vivid details of the incident in which the patient was run over in the street at the age of eight, and the events which appear to have precipitated his illness are also clearly elucidated:

> His present illness dates back for some three years. At that time he fell into a dispute with his dissolute brother, who refused to pay him back a sum of money he had lent him. His brother threatened to stab him and ran at him with a knife. This threw the patient into indescribable fear. (Freud 1886d: 26)

Furthermore, we are told that the patient suffered from headaches, and that the left side of his body never felt quite the same after the incident. Three years later: 'the patient was accused by a woman of a theft, had violent palpitations, was so depressed that he thought of suicide and at the same time a fairly severe tremor set in his left extremities' (Freud 1886d: 27). There follows a detailed clinical demonstration, and then the paper ends with a comment on: 'the characteristic of instability of the disturbance of sensitivity', on the basis of which Freud hopes to: 'restore the patient in a short time to normal sensitivity' (Freud 1886d: 31).

In this case, the question of *history* is opened up for us by Freud; his comments on the events leading up to the development of the patient's symptoms have a quality of high drama which belies Strachey's assertion that the paper contains 'only some very slight indications of interest in psychological factors' (Strachey 1956: 24). In fact, Freud gets us very interested; his words have an almost visual effect, but after he plunges into his clinical description of the patient's anaesthetic symptoms he refers no more to the precipitating events. There is a gap here between history and symptom; something is unexplained. Freud makes absolutely no direct attempt to connect the patient's experiences with his symptom although the connection is implicit.

This question of history shows us a Freud who tolerates his own ignorance. In the subsequent article on hysteria (Freud 1888d) this ignorance is again in evidence. Moreover, Freud admonishes us not to expect to know too much concerning the cause of hysteria. He draws a distinction between anatomy and physiology and, in the process, describes the outlines of a gap in knowledge: 'Not only have no perceptible changes in the nervous system been found in this illness', he informs us, 'but it is not to be expected that any refinement of anatomical techniques would reveal any such changes. Hysteria is based solely and entirely on physiological modifications of the nervous system and its essence should be expressed in a formula which took account of the conditions of excitability in the different parts of the nervous system' (Freud 1888d: 41).

In 'Some Points for a Comparative Study of Organic and Hysterical Motor Paralysis' Freud elaborates upon this, and asserts that '*hysteria behaves as though anatomy did not exist or as though it had no knowledge of it*' (Freud 1893c: 169). Even in 'Sketches for the "Preliminary Communication" of 1893' (Freud 1940-41), in which trauma is connected with hysteria, there remains an ambiguity, something that falls out from this connection. He outlines three groups of hysterical patients: (i) those who 'succumbed to a neurosis after a single major fright'; (ii) those who suffer 'a series of minor [traumas] which are held together by their similarity or by the fact of their forming part of one unhappy story'; and (iii) those whose hysterical attacks 'consist in memories which we should not have judged worthy in themselves of constituting traumas' (Freud 1940-41: 152). It is clear that Freud considers that the observer cannot really judge whether an event is traumatic, but that this is something to do with the subject himself.

In these early writings then, there is a gap in Freud's knowledge about hysteria which he tolerates, and even *encourages* in the reader. It is this unknown that gives these writings their freshness and vivacity. It propels him toward the hysterics and perpetuates his fascination with them. Freud's early encounters with hysteria thus evoke an almost hysterical questioning in *him*. Later, of course, Freud is far more confident in connecting trauma and hysteria. In 'The Aetiology of Hysteria', for instance, he states that: 'there is a... possibility of penetrating from the symptoms to a knowledge of their cause' (Freud 1896c: 192). Eventually, however, this mastery topples over into a lack of knowledge which gives birth to psychoanalysis. Whether this Freudian adventure with hysteria contains a lesson for psychiatry remains to be seen.

Psychiatrists were not quite as plentiful in Freud's time as they are now, so the idea that psychiatry might have constituted a fourth impossible profession did not—perhaps—spring immediately to Freud's mind. However, with its ambitions to become a science of the human subject psychiatry presents, I believe, the ultimate impossibility. It is not difficult to see why this is so, if we examine its current status.

Hippocrates and Galen gave birth to the speciality by attempting to *classify* and *define* mental illnesses. Accurate definition and classification remain the preoccupations of modern psychiatry. The most universally accepted thought in psychiatry is that based on the most rigidly applied scientific methods. It is now relatively difficult to publish an individual psychiatric case history. Whereas, five years ago, one of the most prestigious English language journals carried three or four case histories per issue, we are now lucky to read two a year. We must be 'pure scientists' now; we must have a thorough knowledge of sophisticated statistical methods. As a result a split has emerged between this science of psychiatry and the subject of language with which it is concerned. Psychiatrists assign themselves to the 'organic' or the 'psychotherapeutic' camp, each with its own ethical position, with some professing to be 'eclectic'. This eclecticism operates on its own axioms. In fact, it presents the greatest difficulty by attempting to approach the subject from a scientific perspective while acknowledging the unconscious at an implicit level. This split within the profession of psychiatry is an attempt to deal with the division of the subject of language by identifying oneself with a signifier—'organic', 'psychotherapeutic', or 'eclectic'—and thereafter proceeding as one who is *identified* with this master signifier, thus evading one's own split.

This tension between the neurobiological approach and psychoanalysis is particularly evident in the context of hysteria and trauma. DSM IV, the Diagnostic and Statistical Manual, Fourth Edition, and its UK equivalent, ICD-10, represent the most arid scientific development of a psychiatric body of knowledge, a classification of psychiatric syndromes. The category of hysteria no longer exists in either—it is subsumed under categories such as 'somatisation' or 'somatoform disorder', yet these categories, which reveal the division of the subject so clearly, are fraught with confusion and vagueness. In almost none of the diagnostic categories is there any provision for *aetiology*. The relatively new category of 'post-traumatic stress disorder', which seems to be very similar to the 'traumatic hysteria' of Freud's writings, is the only diagnostic entity for which an aetiology is specified—indeed, it is deemed essential for the diagnosis. While psychoanalysis is not concerned with any linear theory of aetiology, the concept of cause does at least imply the historical. However, the historical view in psychiatry is not the psychoanalytic historical view of a subject who speaks from a place de-centred by history, but—instead—of the *master* who gazes upon the past from a neutral position.

One of the earlier editions (DSM III), specified that for a diagnosis of post-traumatic stress disorder to be made the patient had to have suffered a discrete 'traumatic event' which was 'outside the normal range of human experience'. The observer is, therefore, implicitly instructed to adopt an objective gaze, to decide what was within or outside 'the normal range of experience'—in other words, to adopt a master discourse. Despite this difference in approach to history, the aetiological criterion for the diagnosis of post-traumatic stress disorder does at least imply an existence of history and that the subject speaks about this history. In DSM IV, without wishing to be too optimistic however, it is no longer the experience but the *fear provoked by it* that defines the disorder. This revision suggests a change, albeit not a radical one, in the status of the subject; it suggests *a subject who complains.* Accompanying this alteration in the position of the subject is a change in the status of knowledge about this subject. We cannot know what should or should not be terrifying; this depends only on the subject himself. This revision of DSM does not imply that the profession of psychiatry is abandoning its master position. The confusion that will be evident to anyone who has tried to read the psychiatric discussion on this topic is an effect of *the real,* and the difficulties faced by the authors of DSM are the very crystallisation of the incompleteness of the symbolic order. If the reader has never had the pleasure of examining the abundant literature on the subject of post-traumatic stress disorder, I can assure him or her that it provokes boredom and anxiety. Boredom is a symptom of the attempt to overcome anxiety; the response to this anxiety is predictable—it leads to an attempt to develop a *speciality*. In other words, if we find that what we do not know or understand makes us anxious, we try to become specialists, masters of it. The speciality in this case is called *traumatology,* which must be the epitome of the master discourse, as though one could be a specialist in the divided subject!

One of the more recent treatments devised for traumatised patients is something called 'Eye Movement Desensitisation'. This involves the patient speaking about the traumatic events while following with their eyes the finger movements of the therapist (see Shapiro 1989). That this bears remarkable similarities to hypnosis will be both obvious and amusing to psychoanalysts. The recent surge of interest among psychiatrists in what have been called 'the linguistic therapies' is also quite uncanny, given its striking echoes of the birth of psychoanalysis.

Part of this attempt at mastery is a debate about truth, or about fact. The arguments of Jeffrey Masson concerning Freud's 'abandonment' of the seduction theory are well-known (Masson 1984). From these arguments, which represent a misunderstanding of the signifying nature of memory, there has developed a particularly furious debate regarding 'False Memory Syndrome'. The question asked, in one or another form by those involved in this argument, is 'did it or did it not really happen?' Thus, in response to the insistence of the hysterical division of the subject shown up by any attempts to classify it, to master it, has emerged a discussion concerning the *factual reality* of an incestuous event. This is a logical sequel to the approach of ego psychology. The problem apparently revolves around a question of truth—but it is *'pure, objective truth'* that is in question, not the truth of the unconscious. False Memory Syndrome can only arise in the context of a discursive relationship, but the transference is ignored by a therapist who posits himself as an arbiter of knowledge about the subject. Memory as a *signifying function* is ignored; the real is patched up by an imaginary knowledge about what 'really' happened.

The notion of 'Multiple Personality Disorder' may have a similar origin. Instead of acknowledging the division of the subject, the therapist defines the patient as comprising a multitude of *egos*, each unified in its own right. In the binary science of traumatology, there is little room for the subject whose truth is only in terms of speech. Truth, instead, becomes a matter of objectivity. We *can* know (it is averred) if a frightening event occurred and what reaction to expect—this leads us to a diagnosis of post-traumatic stress disorder. We *can* decide if an event did not occur, disregarding the unconscious—this leads to a diagnosis of false memory syndrome. The furious debate and vast literature created by the problem of trauma bear witness, however, to the insistence of the speaking subject. Such prosaic phenomena as the constant revisions of DSM and the treatments—which may seem ludicrous to psychoanalysts—are all effects of the real that evades science and language and which is central to trauma.

Given the current status of knowledge about hysteria and trauma, it is hardly surprising that psychiatrists feel a certain impotence. Implicit in this study of the vicissitudes of modern psychiatry is a somewhat hysterical question: 'What should psychiatrists *do*?' Just as the hysteric seeks a master, psychiatry erects masters as part of its history, in order to evade the traumatic real. It claims Freud as part of its history, and Freud's early writings in particular are often quoted as proof of the truth of one school of thought or another. For instance, Freud's interest in neuropathology 'proves' that the organic approach is correct, and so on. If we install Freud as the guarantor of truth, the one who 'knew all along' then we imply that the future of our profession has already been determined by its history. This 'necessity' of history has dangers; its results are stagnation of thought, and ideology. To resurrect Freud's early writings on hysteria in order to prove something about psychiatry seems like a search for aetiology.

Instead, I believe we should attempt to rescue the word 'research' from its current connotations. Rather than being a search for cause or determination, research should be literally a *re-search*, an acknowledgement that we cannot know everything about the history of our science or of the hysterical subject to which we address ourselves. Nonetheless when we speak about history we cannot be separated from that speaking, for the place from which we speak is determined in a de-centred way by the real of history. When we look to Freud to articulate something about modern psychiatry, this looking is not with a neutral gaze. Freudian history certainly cannot tell us what we should do or how we should proceed. Hysteria exerted a fascinating effect on Freud and acted as a starting point for analysis, long before Anna O., and hysteria continues to fire our debate and to de-centre our profession.

Perhaps all we can say is that, like Freud, our constantly fluctuating relation to hysteria and to the real are part of the history of hysteria itself. However, Lacan seems to offer a beyond of the inevitability of history:

> What is realised in my history is not the past definite of what was, since it is no more, or even the present perfect of what has been in what I am, but the future anterior of what I shall have been for what I am in the process of becoming. (Lacan 1977b: 86)

If we recognise in our own experience with hysteria a repetition of Freud's trajectory from ignorance to mastery, and back again, then we must also take account of the real that is bound up with that repetition. (It must also be remembered that Freud himself did not always maintain this *docta ignorantia*, as we can see in the case of Dora [Freud 1905d].) This may not necessarily allow us to articulate an ethical position for psychiatry—which is clearly quite unlike psychoanalysis. However, this history may confront us with our unavoidable ignorance concerning hysteria which—thankfully—makes a position of mastery untenable.

Notes

[1] The restiform nucleus, also known as the inferior cerebellar peduncle, carries nerve fibres from the spinocerebellar tracts to the cerebellum, and is thus involved in the control of balance and movement. See Chusid 1985.

PSYCHIC DETERMINATION IN NEUROSIS: ON THE ROLE OF CONSTITUTION IN EARLY FREUDIAN THEORY

Katrien Libbrecht

Introduction

In Lecture 18 of the *Introductory Lectures on Psychoanalysis*, 'Fixation to Traumas—The Unconscious', Freud writes:

> these symptoms [of obsessional neurosis] offer the plainest indication of there being a special region of the mind, shut off from the rest. They lead, by a path that cannot be missed, to a conviction of the existence of the unconscious in the mind; and that is precisely why clinical psychiatry, which is acquainted only with a psychology of consciousness, can deal with these symptoms in no other way than by declaring them to be signs of a special sort of degeneracy. (Freud 1916-17: 278)

I have chosen this passage because it shows that, in 1915, Freud argued that the hypothesis of the unconscious counters the psychiatric notion of degeneracy and supersedes its explanatory value. Put more concretely, Freud demonstrates that the existence of the unconscious and of unconscious psychic processes make it possible to explain psychically and elucidate so-called consciously inexplicable symptoms. In this sense, the hypothesis of the unconscious, which implies a psychic explanation and determination of neurotic symptoms, renders redundant the notion of degeneracy, which involves a constitutional and hereditary determination of neurotic symptoms. Hence, we could say that Freud's notion of the unconscious implies that neurotic symptoms, and more generally neurosis as such, can—indeed, must—be explained without calling upon some constitutional, non-psychic element. Thus, we could conclude that the notion of the unconscious implies the idea of psychic causality.

At this point, two questions arise: (i) Does the notion of the unconscious psychic determination of neurotic symptoms mean that Freud proclaims a purely psychodeterminist view of mental functioning? (ii) Is it necessary, in this respect, to distinguish between Freud's early theorisations on the aetiology of neurosis—that is, those stemming from the period of Freud's so-called pre-analytic works written from before 1900—and his later writings on this subject?

I will try to formulate an answer to these questions by studying Freud's early aetiological theory on neurosis, and sketching its subsequent evolution.

Charcot's Influence on early Freudian Theory

It is well known that, in October 1885, Freud went to study with Jean-Martin Charcot at the Salpêtrière in Paris. Upon his return to Vienna, in March 1886, Freud proclaimed himself a disciple of Charcot. His request to translate one of the volumes of Charcot's lessons into German can be considered as one of the first concrete indications of Freud's fascination and respect for the figure and the teachings of the Master. Additional and, to me, more interesting indications of this transference onto Charcot can be found in several of Freud's writings dating from the period following his stay in Paris. These articles are more interesting because they reflect Freud's scientific struggle with Charcotian ideas.

For evidence of this, we can refer to the following: Freud's first article on hysteria entitled 'Observation of a Severe Case of Hemi-Anesthesia in a Hysterical Male' (Freud 1886d); his article 'Hysteria' (Freud 1888d) which appeared in the Villaret encyclopaedia; the French article 'Quelques considérations pour une étude comparative des paralysies motrices organiques et hystériques' (translated as Freud 1893c); and 'On the Psychical Mechanism of Hysterical Phenomena' (Freud 1893e). All of these writings demonstrate how and to what extent early Freudian theory on psychopathology was influenced by the ideas of Charcot. In this respect, a less remarkable, though highly instructive article is *'L'hérédité et l'étiologie des névroses'* (translated as Freud 1896a), which presents a most explicit and critical evaluation of Charcot's aetiological theory on neurosis, and places nervous heredity (*hérédité nerveuse*) centre stage.

Freud's encounter with Charcot is generally seen as a confrontation with Charcot's experimental—and by no means therapeutic—use of hypnotic suggestion. It is also claimed that this encounter led Freud to a major turn in his scientific career, namely the shift from neurology to psychopathology. However, this is the full extent to which Charcot's role in Freud's discovery of the unconscious and his development of psychoanalytic theory is attributed. To put it more bluntly, the study of the influence of Charcot's theorisations on Freud has, thus far, not been fully exploited. One way, for instance, in which Charcot's work was clearly influential on Freud's thinking, is his view on the formative role the idea plays in the formation of the hysterical picture. Charcot discovered this through his study of hystero-traumatic paralyses—for instance, the fact that the autosuggestive idea of being paralysed produces a hysterical paralysis (Micale 1994). Here, the famous Freudian phrase 'hysteria suffers from reminiscences' easily falls into place. Another aspect of Charcot's influence, which I have developed elsewhere, concerns the notion of psychic trauma, which is present in Charcot's studies of male hysteria or hystérie virile (Libbrecht & Quackelbeen 1995).

This chapter—however—deals with yet another aspect of Charcot's theory. Departing from a reading of *'L'hérédité et l'étiologie des névroses'*, I shall demonstrate how Freud, in the style of a critical dialogue, positions his theory on the aetiology of neurosis in general—and of hysteria in particular—within the more general debate on the role of constitution in the aetiology of neurosis. Hence, the element I shall focus on is the place reserved for the aetiological role of (hereditary) constitution, an element which Freud explicitly refers to in this text, but which seems either forgotten or overlooked in considerations of Freud's psychoanalytic writings.

Freud versus Charcot on Neuropathic Heredity

'L'hérédité et l'étiologie des névroses' was published in 1896, when Freud was developing his theory on the notion of psychic defence (*Abwehr*), on the basis of which he characterised and distinguished between various neuropsychoses of defence. The texts which are usually considered in this context are the *Studies on Hysteria*, and Freud's two papers on the neuropsychoses of defence (Breuer & Freud 1895; Freud 1894, 1896b). Although the notion of psychic defence is crucial in Freud's theorisations on symptom formation, putting a psychic mechanism centre stage does not a priori imply a psychic aetiological reasoning. Indeed, Charcot also eventually took into account the operation of a psychic mechanism in order to explain the symptom formation in hysteria, but never abandoned his aetiological theory in which the role of heredity (*l'hérédité nerveuse*) predominated.

In 'On the Psychical Mechanism of Hysterical Phenomena: Preliminary Communication', the first chapter of the Studies on Hysteria, we read:

> If by uncovering the psychical mechanism of hysterical phenomena we have taken a step forward along the path first traced so successfully by Charcot with his explanation and artificial imitation of hystero-traumatic paralyses, we cannot conceal from ourselves that this has brought us nearer to an understanding only of the mechanism of hysterical symptoms and not of the internal causes of hysteria. We have done no more than touch upon the aetiology of hysteria and have been able to throw light only on its acquired forms—on the bearing of accidental factors of the neurosis. (Breuer & Freud 1893: 17)

Thus, according to Freud, the psychic mechanism of defence only touches upon the accidental factors of neurosis and does not account for its internal causes. In that case, what are these internal causes?

An appropriate way to study Freud's aetiological theory on neurosis, and more particularly on the neuropsychoses of defence, is to examine the questions which were haunting him in the 1890s, of which the article *'L'hérédité et l'étiologie des névroses'* draws a fairly clear picture. At this stage Freud touches upon three fundamental questions concerning the aetiology of neurosis:

(i). What determines the choice of neurosis, ie., the particular type of neurosis? Here, the notion of *étiologie spécifique* is introduced.

(ii). How can one account for the fact that a specific aetiological influence does not cause the same neurotic or pathological effect in each subject? At this point Freud mentions the role of heredity as being a disposition or precondition to neurosis determining the pathological response.

(iii). What triggers the onset of neurosis, ie., what renders the neurosis manifest? Here, Freud refers to Charcot's notion of *agent provocateur*.

Freud's article can be interpreted in different ways. The most obvious and most common reading is that Freud introduces the new aetiological element of the *sexual* cause of the neuroses, and thereby substitutes the Charcotian notion of neuropathic constitution with the role of sexuality. Sexuality could then, in turn, provide the answer to Freud's questioning of the internal causes of hysteria.

My reading, however, starts with the way in which Freud positions his own findings within the frame of Charcot's aetiological theory and thereby calls into question the role of the constitutional factor.

Freud starts off with a thorough critique, comprising six arguments, of the role of the so-called neuropathic constitution in the determination of the *névropathies*. He ends the first section of his article by introducing the question of *specific aetiology*, which is, in his view, far more important than the question of heredity, since the latter cannot come into play without the presence of a specific cause, which accounts for the specificity of the affection.

Only in the second section of his article does Freud enter into the question of the aetiology of the neuroses, characterised as 'functional nervous states analogous to hysteria' (Freud 1896a: 146). Concurrent with the three aforementioned aetiological questions, Freud distinguishes between three kinds of aetiological influences on neurosis (comprising both the 'psychoneuroses' and what Freud will later call *Aktualneurosen*). These aetiological influences include:

(i). Preconditions or necessary conditions, which are not specific to a particular kind of neurosis; here, Freud stresses the role of *heredity* as a disposition or precondition to neurosis.

(ii). The concurrent, non-specific causes, which are of universal nature, but are not essential for neurotic pathology. This is the set of *agents provocateurs*, which triggers the onset of neurosis.[1]

(iii). The necessary, specific causes, determining the nature of the neurosis. We already indicated that this third class of influences constitutes a new element with regard to Charcot's aetiological theory.

What can be inferred from this? Firstly, according to Freud in this article, heredity as a disposition is responsible for the fact that, given a specific aetiological influence, one subject develops neurosis whereas another does not. In other words, in Freud's view, heredity can account for or explain the pathological neurotic response.

He compares the influence of a hereditary disposition to that of the 'multiplier' in an electric circuit. The multiplier amplifies the visible deviation of the needle but, by itself, it is not capable of determining its direction. To Freud, who refers to the question of *Neurosenwahl,* the direction pathology takes is determined by the *specific* cause, which—he argues in this article—resides within the realm of sexuality. Neurosis, therefore, is either due to a disturbance of the present sexual life, or originates from important events in the past—that is, in the sexual life history. For hysteria, this is identified as a premature, passive sexual experience.

Secondly, and this refines the first conclusion, Freud's text makes it quite clear that the specific sexual cause is of major importance to him. It represents his most innovatory idea on aetiology. It was not the discovery of the role of sexuality as such that was new at the time—the influence of sexuality had already been discussed by various other authors—but rather Freud's accentuation of the impact and the function of sexuality in the determination of neurosis:

> What gives its distinctive character to my line of approach is that I elevate these sexual influences to the rank of specific causes, that I recognise their action in every case of neurosis, and finally that I trace a regular parallelism, a proof of a specific aetiological relation between the nature of the sexual influence and the pathological species of the neurosis. (Freud 1896a: 149)

Freud argues that the aetiological influence of sexuality had always been restricted to a limited number of cases, subordinated to the influence of heredity, and inscribed within the large set of *agents provocateurs*. In addition to this, Freud's elaboration shows that sexuality as a specific cause is the only truly essential one. For, as we already mentioned, without this aetiological influence, heredity cannot come into play. What is more, in cases of so-called 'acquired neurosis', the hereditary factor proves absent. This is also implicitly invoked by Freud in his remark concerning the relative quantities of the aetiological influences, meaning that heredity and specific causes can substitute one another in a quantitative way. For instance, this implies that the same pathological effect can be produced by the concurrence of a serious specific aetiology and a moderate disposition, or perhaps by a severe nervous heredity and a minor specific influence. Freud stresses that in some cases no hereditary influence is to be traced, but does not argue the same for the specific aetiological factor. Hence our conclusion that Freud considers only one important aetiological factor: *sexuality*. We should add to this that Freud emphasises the practical, psychotherapeutic value of the specific cause, whereas if one privileges the notion of hereditary constitution, one highlights the limits of psychotherapeutic and/or psychoanalytic work.

I argued that Freud's article presents a critical evaluation of Charcot's aetiological theory on neurosis, which places nervous heredity (*hérédité nerveuse*) centre stage. The first major contribution Freud makes, then, is that sexuality plays an essential aetiological role in all cases of neurosis, insofar as it determines the direction pathology takes. Secondly, Freud argues that the premature sexual experience is a major causal factor, especially in cases of psychoneurosis and thus particularly in cases of hysteria. Along the same lines, Freud argues that, in cases of psychoneurosis, the premature sexual experience occupies the same aetiological place as nervous heredity does within Charcot's aetiological theory. What this means, then, is that the *psychic* determination of neurosis is dominant in cases of psychoneuroses. However, it does not mean that the factor of heredity is radically excluded in all of these cases; it is only absent in cases of acquired neurosis. Hence, Freud indicates that Charcot's theory formally and unjustly neglects the major aetiological influence of sexuality.

Hysterical Symptoms versus Hysteria

The next question we shall consider is whether these conclusions tally with Freud's other writings from the same period, and more particularly with those writings which do not explicitly refer to Charcot's theory.

Let us first turn to the *Studies on Hysteria*. It is evident from the case studies under discussion here that Freud's primary concern is to demonstrate how hysterical symptoms are psychically determined. Furthermore, it is evident that it is Freud's therapeutic concern or desire that leads him to question the basic element of hysterical symptom formation—namely, the splitting of consciousness due to an incompatible idea or trauma—and more particularly to discover the psychic mechanism of the conversion of an excitation into a somatic innervation. As far as the aetiology of hysteria as a pathological response is concerned, we learn that, here too, Freud invokes some kind of hereditary constitution, which acts as a general disposition.

For instance, in his discussion of the case of Emmy von N., he writes:

> Frau von N. was undoubtedly a personality with a severe neuropathic heredity. It seems likely that there can be no hysteria apart from a disposition of this kind. But on the other hand disposition alone does not make hysteria. There must be reasons that bring it about, and, in my opinion, these reasons must be appropriate: the aetiology is of a specific character. (Breuer & Freud 1895: 102).

Thus heredity, as a disposition, seems responsible for Emmy's pathological response, although heredity alone cannot account for (the choice of) hysteria as such. A third question which surfaces in the discussion of Emmy concerns the onset of hysteria:

> I am now of the opinion that there must have been some added factor to provoke the outbreak of illness precisely in these last years, considering that operative aetiological conditions had been present for many years previously. (Breuer & Freud 1895: 102-103)

Hence, as far as this case of hysteria is concerned, we could conclude that Freud indeed considers three kinds of aetiological influences.

In his discussion of the case of Miss Lucy R., characterised as a case of slight and mild hysteria, Freud argues:

> I am tempted to regard it as a model instance of one particular type of hysteria, namely the form of this illness which can be acquired even by a person of sound heredity, as a result of appropriate experiences. (Breuer & Freud 1895: 122)

In the light of our discussion of Freud's 1896 article, one could argue that, in this case, there is no question of a hereditary or constitutional influence. But Freud proceeds:

> It should be understood that I do not mean by this a hysteria which is independent of any pre-existing disposition. It is probable that no such hysteria exists... A neuropathic disposition... is something different... Her hysteria can... be described as an acquired one, and it presupposed nothing more than the possession of what is probably a widespread proclivity—the proclivity to acquire hysteria. We have as yet scarcely a notion of what the features of this proclivity may be. In cases of this kind, however, the main emphasis falls upon the nature of the trauma, though taken in conjunction of course, with the subject's reaction to it. (Breuer & Freud 1895: 122)

From this, therefore, we can infer that Freud distinguishes between at least two different kinds of disposition, a *general* one and a *specific* one. As well as the general (Charcotian) neuropathic heredity, which is absent in the case of Lucy R., Freud indicates the presence of a specific disposition, defined here as the proclivity to acquire hysteria. This leads us to the conclusion that Freud believes that an element of disposition is essential for all cases of hysteria, including the acquired forms. Is this what Freud is referring to in the 'Preliminary Communication' when he speaks of the internal causes of hysteria which are not of an accidental nature? This would imply that disposition, connected to the specific cause, is of a constitutional rather than of an accidental nature.

Before developing this point a little further, let us first pause on these notions of 'constitution' and 'accident'. In his article on heredity and aetiology, Freud distinguished between three classes of aetiological influences, based on what could be called the variables of necessity and specificity.[2] In addition, the *Studies on Hysteria* makes clear that Freud also uses another, dual aetiological reasoning which takes into consideration the influence of constitution and accident. This dual model can hardly be called typical of Freud's reasoning, for it does not convey any of the particularities of his view. Charcot, for instance, also used this dual aetiological model of constitution versus accident. However, the difference between Freud's and Charcot's view reflects their views on the role of sexuality, and implies that this interpretation of duality is characteristic of Freud's reasoning.

Let us start with Charcot's interpretation, specified by Freud as follows:

> in the view of the influential school of Charcot, heredity alone deserves to be recognised as the true cause of hysteria, while all other noxae of the most various nature and intensity only play the part of incidental causes, of *'agents provocateurs'*. (Freud 1896c: 191)

Freud's interpretation, for which he makes use of the variables of necessity and specificity, can be read as the opposite of Charcot's. For, in contrast to Charcot, Freud does not consider a hereditary constitution to be essential in all cases of neurosis, although it is 'powerful in every case and indispensable in most cases' (Freud 1896a: 147). The only truly necessary element is the so-called accidental factor of sexuality, which is present in *all* cases of hysteria, and which accounts for the symptoms. To complete the picture, Freud also takes into account the accidental factor of the concurrent causes, which trigger the onset of neurosis.

From the above we could conclude that in the mid 1890s, and in contrast to the prevailing medical opinion, Freud considers the *accidental* factor of prime importance in the determination of neurosis. However, our discussion of the case of Lucy R. did raise another suggestion on the matter, for it seems that in *Studies on Hysteria* Freud reintroduces the element of constitution on the level of specific aetiology by means of the notion of 'proclivity'. Indeed, the question which Freud's discussion of Lucy R. raises, concerns the nature of the specific (sexual) cause: is this specific cause only accidental in nature, or does it also comprise a constitutional element? If the latter were the case, this would lead us to the conclusion that Freud considers both (sexual) constitution and (sexual) accident as conditions for the development of neurosis.

Hereditary Constitution versus Sexual Constitution

In the article 'Further Remarks on the Neuro-Psychoses of Defence', Freud speaks of the specific cause in terms of an accidental aetiological factor:

> I have found this specific determinant of hysteria—*sexual passivity during the pre-sexual period*—in every case of hysteria (including two male cases) which I have analysed. How greatly the claims of hereditary disposition are diminished by the establish-

> ment in this way of accidental aetiological factors as a determinant needs no more than a mention (Freud 1896b: 163).

However, Freud's subsequent writings on the role of sexuality in neurosis indicate that he indeed reformulates the question of hereditary constitution in terms of sexual constitution, thereby introducing constitution on the level of the specific cause. For instance, in the article 'My Views on the Part Played by Sexuality in the Aetiology of the Neuroses', we read:

> Along with the supposed frequency of seduction in childhood, I ceased also to lay exaggerated stress on the *accidental* influencing of sexuality on to which I had sought to thrust the main responsibility for the causation of the illness, though I had not on that account denied the constitutional and hereditary factors... Accidental influences derived from experience having thus receded into the background, the factors of constitution and heredity necessarily gained the upper hand once more; but there was this difference between my views and those prevailing in other quarters, that on my theory the 'sexual constitution' took the place of a 'general neuropathic disposition'. (Freud 1906: 275-276)

The following excerpt from 'On the History of the Psychoanalytic Movement' can be read in a similar way:

> With this sexual activity of the first years of childhood the inherited constitution of the individual also came into its own. Disposition and experience are here linked up in an indissoluble aetiological unity. For *disposition* exaggerates impressions which would otherwise have been completely commonplace and have had no effect, so that they become traumas giving rise to stimulations and fixations; while *experiences* awaken factors in the disposition which, without them, might have long remained dormant and perhaps never have developed. The last word on the subject of traumatic aetiology was spoken later by Abraham (1907), when he pointed out that the sexual constitution which is peculiar to children is precisely calculated to provoke sexual experiences of a particular kind—namely traumas. (Freud 1914: 18)

These passages indicate that, in Freud's view, the element of constitution and of accident eventually share the major characteristic of being sexual in nature. In other terms, Freud adheres to his basic notion of a specific sexual cause, though it comprises both constitutional and accidental elements: 'disposition and experience are here linked up in an indissoluble aetiological unity'. In his 1912 article on 'The Dynamics of Transference', Freud coined this dual aetiological influence as the principle of 'Endowment' and 'Chance':

> I take this opportunity of defending myself against the mistaken charge of having denied the importance of innate (constitutional) factors because I have stressed that of infantile impressions... Psychoanalysis has talked a lot about the accidental factors in aetiology and little about the constitutional ones; but that is only because it was able to contribute something fresh to the former, while, to begin with, it knew no more than was commonly known about the latter... 'Δαιμων και Τυχη' [Endowment and Chance] determine a man's fate—rarely or never one of these powers alone. The amount of aetiological effectiveness to be attributed to each of them can only be arrived at in every individual case separately. (Freud 1912: 99)

A similar statement can be read in Freud's lecture 'Transference'.[3] In the light of what we have developed, this should not be surprising at all, since the transference is the motor of the psychoanalytic process and by the same token also of therapeutic effectiveness. In this sense, it is essential for Freud to articulate the constitutional limits in which psychoanalysis is bound to work.[4]

A small passage at the end of the footnote on Endowment and Chance, in 'The Dynamics of Transference', gives an additional hint for the interpretation of Endowment, or the constitutional part: 'Incidentally, one might venture to regard constitution itself as a precipitate from the accidental effects produced on the endlessly long chain of our ancestors' (Freud 1912: 99).[5] In view of the ideas in this chapter, this could be read in the following way: human sexuality by its very nature is traumatic and is the sole cause of neurotic pathology.

Conclusion and Implications

The first conclusion we can draw from our study of Freud's early aetiological theory of neurosis, is that the influence of hereditary constitution is far more important than we initially thought and than is generally accepted. It became clear how Freud, after firstly heavily criticising the notion of neuropathic constitution, reintroduced constitution as an essential element of neurosis by linking it to sexuality as a specific cause. Hereditary constitution was replaced by sexual constitution as a 'prehistoric experience'. Furthermore, since the constitutional element is at no point specified by Freud as being purely psychic in nature—Freud does not actually say much about the constitutional factor in general—we can argue that his early aetiological theory of neurosis does not unequivocally testify to a psychodeterminist point of view. Indeed, much depends on how the element of constitution is interpreted. Moreover, since Freud links constitution to sexuality, it would be more appropriate to speak of a *sexual determinism*, thereby introducing the new question of how the sexual and the psychic are both interrelated and appreciated in Freud's (early) view. In my opinion, the introduction of the notion of 'psychosexuality' does not really solve the matter, since this cannot account for what Freud called the '*Aktualneurosen*'.

The second point we discussed, namely that Freud definitely uses a dual aetiological reasoning, which is composed of a constitutional or innate and an accidental factor, both of which are sexual in nature, renders this questioning even more necessary, and reopens rather than closes the debate concerning the notion of '(psychic) causality' within early psychoanalytic theory. In this sense, it is important to bear in mind that, in subsequent works, particularly in the passage of his article on transference, Freud writes that he did not abandon his dual aetiological model and also explicitly states why he did not further investigate the part played by 'Endowment', but instead concentrated his efforts on 'Chance'—that is, the accidental, psychic and/or sexual factor. Furthermore, the part played by the constitutional element sheds a different light on Freud's notion of the 'curability' of neurosis and on the therapeutic effectiveness of psychoanalysis.[6]

Let us come back to our two initial questions, the first of which asked whether the notion of an unconscious psychic determination of neurotic symptoms entails that Freud proclaims a purely psychodeterminist view of mental functioning. I concluded that the answer to this question implies an interpretation of the notion of constitution in Freud's theory, and that it is not adequate to interpret this as purely psychic in nature. Moreover, although Freud believes that unconscious psychic determination is the only matter psychoanalysis can work with, the limits set by constitution determine the extent of change which is possible and, in this sense, constitution is indeed relevant as far as the (potential) *treatment* of neurosis is concerned. My second question was whether it was necessary, in this respect, to distinguish between what is referred to as the period of Freud's pre-analytic writings and the period of the so-called analytic writings. We can now answer this question in two ways. Firstly, in a negative way: Freud persisted in taking into account the role of constitution, even though this shifted from hereditary (neuropathic) constitution to (hereditary) sexual constitution. Secondly, in an affirmative way: Freud's discovery of unconscious processes—which, for instance, is already clear in the *Studies on Hysteria*—is the primary cause of his critique of Charcot's aetiological theory, which placed nervous hereditary disposition centre stage, and to which Freud, at least initially, subscribed.

Notes

1 These concurrent influences include all kinds of trivial agents—for example: moral emotions, traumatic accidents, somatic exhaustion, acute illness, intoxication and intellectual overflow. Although these agents are regularly present and not necessary for the development of neurosis, Freud does consider them of value. For one, these banal agents are always invoked by patients to explain their suffering and can trigger the onset of neurosis. These *agents provocateurs* render manifest a hitherto latent neurosis. Furthermore, Freud adds the interesting remark that these banal causes are also of therapeutic value, in case one does not opt for a radical treatment, but chooses for a repression of the disorder to its former state of latency. Hence, Freud differentiates between what could be called a kind of rehabilitative psychotherapy and psychoanalysis.

2 Indeed, Freud distinguished between preconditions, concurrent causes and specific causes, which he characterised respectively as: indispensable and of a general nature, dispensable and of a general nature, and indispensable and of a specific nature.

3 It concerns the following passage: 'Think it over! You have learnt all that is essential about the determinants of falling ill as well as all the factors that come into effect *after* the patient has fallen ill. Where do these leave room for any therapeutic influence? In the first place there is hereditary disposition. We have not talked about it very often because it is emphatically stressed from other directions and we have nothing new to say about it. But do not suppose that we under-estimate it; precisely as therapists we come to realise its power clearly enough. In any case we can do nothing to alter it; we too must take it as something given, which sets a limit to our efforts' (Freud 1916-17: 431-432).

4 The idea that constitution indicates the limits of curability can also be found in other papers on technique (Freud 1904; 1905a) and, for instance, in the lecture 'Explanations, Applications and Orientations' (Freud 1933: 153-154).

5 This idea of constitutional disposition (heredity) as an after-effect of 'experiences by ancestors in the past' is further developed in Introductory Lecture 23, 'Paths of the Formation of Symptoms' (Freud 1916-17: 361-362).

6 Freud's final elaborations—from the 1920s—indicate that he links heredity to the *Id* and to culture (see Freud 1923: 38). In this sense, a close investigation of Freud's later writings might reveal that his dual model eventually comprised the constitutional element of culture and cultural inheritance on the one hand, and the accidental factor of life-history on the other. A detailed study of the evolution of the notion of constitution and heredity in the works of Freud might establish that, eventually, Freudian theory stressed the *cultural* element as determinative in psychic functioning.

'MY BAD DIAGNOSTIC ERROR': RE-VISITING THE CASE OF EMMY VON N. (FANNY MOSER)

Christfried Tögel

The first case presented by Freud in *Studies on Hysteria* is that of Emmy von N. He wrote:

> On May 1, 1889, I took on the case of a lady of about forty years of age, whose symptoms and personality interested me so greatly that I devoted a large part of my time to her and determined to do all I could for her recovery. (Breuer & Freud 1895: 48)

In 1960 the evident importance of this case in the early history of psychoanalysis led Kurt Eissler, of the Sigmund Freud Archives in New York, to ask Ola Andersson from Stockholm to undertake further research about Emmy von N. and, hopefully, to discover her identity.[1]

Having spent a lot of time on research, and having travelled for some weeks in Switzerland and Austria, Andersson presented Eissler with some quite impressive results. He was able to inform him of the real name of Emmy von N., and to provide other biographical details.

In 1965, at the International Psychoanalytic Congress in Amsterdam, Andersson read a paper in which he presented some of his findings, but without revealing the identity of Freud's patient (Andersson, 1979). It was not until the 1970s that two articles identifying Emmy von N. were published: one by Karl Schib, a historian from Schaffhausen, the home town of Emmy's husband (Schib, 1970); and another by Henri Ellenberger, the great historian of psychiatry (Ellenberger, 1977). Since then there have been no developments.

Last year, however, while working at the Sigmund Freud Archives in the Library of Congress, I came across an unpublished letter from Freud to a certain 'Frau Doktor' (Freud 1935a). This letter was filed under the supposed addressee—Gerda Walther, a German parapsychologist. It might be supposed that she had written to Freud, and that the letter was Freud's reply. However, the actual content of the letter made me suspicious. After having read it thoroughly, I became convinced that this 'Frau Doktor' was not Gerda Walther, but—in fact—the eldest daughter of Freud's famous patient, 'Emmy von N.'

Since I was already interested in Freud's early cases, and in determining the exact dates of their treatment, I put together all the available information on Emmy von N., based on the following sources: Freud's account of the treatment in the *Studies on Hysteria* (Breuer & Freud 1895: 48-105); Andersson's and Ellenberger's research on the biographical background of Emmy von N. (Andersson 1979: 7, 1960, 1962a); and the letter I found in the Library of Congress, and my own research concerning the dating of the case (Tögel 1994: 134-136; Freud 1935a).

Using these sources, I will briefly outline Emmy von N.'s case.

Emmy von N. was referred to Freud by Josef Breuer. She displayed the following symptoms, most of which arose after her husband's death, fourteen years previously: from time to time her speech was subject to spastic interruptions like a stammer; she displayed frequent convulsive tic-like movements of her face; she frequently interrupted her remarks by producing a curious 'clacking' sound from her mouth. In addition, every two or three minutes she suddenly broke off, contorted her face into an expression of horror and disgust, stretched out her hand towards Freud, spreading and crooking her fingers, and exclaimed in a changed voice charged with anxiety: 'Keep still! Don't say anything!—Don't touch me!'

Freud summarised the psychical situation of Emmy von N. in two basic points: firstly, that the distressing affects connected to her traumatic experiences had remained unresolved; and secondly that her memory was gradually bringing her traumas and their accompanying affects into her present-day consciousness.

Freud described the treatment and its success as follows:

> My therapeutic procedure was based on the course of this activity of her memory and endeavoured day by day to resolve and get rid of whatever that particular day had brought to the surface, till the accessible stock of her pathological memories seemed to be exhausted... The therapeutic success on the whole was considerable; but it was not a lasting one. (Breuer & Freud 1895: 90-101)

So—who was Emmy von N. and what do we know about her life and family? Ola Andersson was the first person to discover her real identity, and reported his results in as yet unpublished letters to Kurt Eissler. His research was completed by Ellenberger. Today we know that Emmy von N. was born on 28th July, 1848, as Fanny Louise von Sulzer-Wart. At the age of 22 she married Heinrich Moser, a very wealthy Swiss industrialist, a manufacturer of watches. He was 44 years older than Fanny, and died four years after their wedding. The couple had two children: Fanny, born in 1872; and Mentona, born 1874, three days before the death of her father. Shortly after her husband's death, Fanny—the mother—began to develop her symptoms and underwent treatment in different European spas.

At this point, I would like to make some comments on the dating of the Fanny Moser's case. All attempts to date the treatment of Fanny Moser consistently failed, as did the chronology in the appendix of the English translation of the *Studies on Hysteria* in the *Standard Edition* (Breuer & Freud 1895: 307-309), as well as the datings of Henri Ellenberger (1977) and Ola Andersson (1979). Problems arose because of Freud's confusing account of the timetable of the treatment. Freud usually altered *several* circumstances of the case, in order to hide the identity of his patient—for example her name and her residence. The question is, whether he changed the dates of the treatment as well. Ellenberger and Andersson eventually came to the conclusion that the treatment began on 1st May, 1889—that is, Freud stated it correctly. There is no reason to believe that Freud altered the age of Fanny's daughters in order to make the identification of his patient more difficult, as was assumed by Appignanesi & Forrester (1992: 490). Therefore we can conclude that he did indeed reveal the correct dates of the treatment, despite the fact that—in at least two other cases in the *Studies on Hysteria*—he altered them (as in the case of Ilona Weiss, alias 'Elisabeth von R.') or left them undecided (as in the case of 'Katharina').

If we try to put together all the information about the case of Fanny Moser, and the circumstances of Freud's life in the period from 1888 until 1891, we are able to date the treatment without any contradictions. This timetable reads as follows:

- In mid-March 1888, Fanny Moser came to Vienna in order to be treated by Josef Breuer. Freud took over the case on May 1 and treated her for seven weeks, until 17th June, 1888.

- One year later, at the end of April 1889, Fanny returned to Vienna for a second course of treatment by Freud. It lasted eight weeks, until 21st June, 1889.

- Four weeks later, on 19th July, 1889, Freud visited her in Au, near Zürich, on his way to Nancy and Paris.

- The next year, in May 1890, Freud was asked by Fanny Moser to give his opinion on the condition of Fanny's eldest daughter, and he visited her again at her estate in Switzerland.

This dating is confirmed by the following fact: Freud reports that, during the first course of the treatment, Fanny Moser read about the outbreak of a revolution in San Domingo, and was very concerned because one of her brothers lived there. However, Fanny Moser's brother did not emigrate to San Domingo (as Freud states) but to Haiti (see Ellenberger 1993: 280; Denzler 1933). Therefore the revolution in question took place not in San Domingo, but in Haiti. In actual fact: 'Civil war was waged in 1888-89 between Generals Légitime and Hippolyte, and the latter succeeded in obtaining the vacant presidency' (The Encyclopaedia Britannica 1910: 826).

The only point which needs some explanation is the fact that Fanny Moser's younger daughter, Mentona, mentions in her unpublished autobiography that her mother heard of the double-suicide of Kronprinz Rudolf and Mary Vetsera in Mayerling during her stay in the spa of Abbazia, before going to Vienna—that is, in January 1889 (cf. Andersson 1979: 12). However, there is no reason to assume that this stay in Abbazia was the *first* for Fanny Moser and her daughters. Evidently, they had been in Abbazia not only in the winter of 1888/1889, but in the previous winter as well. This is in accordance to Freud's account of their stay in Abbazia before the first course of treatment, and does not contradict Mentona Moser's account in her autobiography, which refers to another stay one year later.

I will now return to the case itself. As I have already mentioned, in May 1890 Fanny Moser asked Freud to give his opinion on the condition of her eldest daughter, who became more and more estranged from her mother. Freud agreed and after a stay of few days in Au he concluded that the daughter had:

> ...entered on a phase of abnormal development. She exhibited unbridled ambitions which were out of all proportions to the poverty of her gifts, and she became disobedient and even violent towards her mother. (Breuer & Freud 1895: 83)

At this point, I shall refer to the letter I uncovered, from Freud to Fanny's daughter, dated 1935. The most important part of this letter reads:

> I cannot blame you that you still haven't forgiven my bad diagnostic error at that time. I was not only inexperienced, but our skills in reading the hidden psyche were still in their infancy. Ten, maybe five years later, I couldn't have helped guessing that the unlucky woman fought a serious battle against the unconscious hatred for her two children and tried to defend herself by means of over-tenderness. These evil ghosts seemed to have reached the surface and determined her behaviour. But at that time I didn't understand anything and just believed in her information. (Freud 1935a)[2]

Thus, in the letter, Freud revises the diagnosis he made half a century previously, qualifying it as 'a bad diagnostic error', and apologising to the daughter.

Why did Freud initially come to this unfavourable conclusion, and why did he revise it decades later?[3] The answer to the first part of this question lies—as Freud himself suggests—in the level of his therapeutic skills in the 1880s and 1890s. At this time, Freud quite naively believed almost everything his patients told him. For instance, at the end of his account of Emmy von N. in the *Studies on Hysteria*, Freud characterises Fanny as follows:

> The woman we came to know was an admirable one. The moral seriousness with which she viewed her duties, her intelligence and energy, which were no less than a man's, and her high degree of education and love of truth impressed both of us greatly; while her benevolent care for the welfare of all her dependents, her humility of mind and the refinement of her manners revealed her qualities as a true lady as well. (Breuer & Freud 1895: 103-4)

He also comments that her attempts at suppressing her sexual needs had exposed her to severe mental exhaustion.

In contrast, the information Andersson and Ellenberger gathered on Fanny Moser paints a quite different picture. Andersson writes:

> ...she nearly always seems to have had lovers and erotic relationships, sometimes with doctors whom she consulted at the spas, or who lived in her house as her personal doctors... they were in sharp contrast to the air of moral earnestness, which impressed several visitors as a prominent trait of her character... (Andersson 1979: 11)

Evidently, one of the people 'impressed' in this way was Sigmund Freud.

It seems that, later, he changed his mind regarding the personality of Fanny Moser junior for two principal reasons. Firstly, Freud's contact with Fanny Moser junior lasted more than 40 years. He knew about her scientific career as a zoologist (cf. Moser 1925) and occasionally received letters from her. (One of his replies, from 1918, was partially published in Andersson 1979: 15.) In 1935 she sent him her latest work, a study on occultism in two volumes (Moser 1935). At the end of his letter to her, Freud comments:

> I have read some paragraphs of your book. I appreciate it as a brave and honest deed, one step further on the most stony path of work. You won't be surprised that I can't agree entirely with the pure theoretical chapters on hypnotism, dream, hysteria, especially with that on 'subconscious'. (Freud 1935a)[4]

The second reason for his change of opinion was that, over the years, Freud became more and more experienced in interpreting the information he obtained from his patients. As he puts it in his letter: '...at that time I didn't understand anything and just believed in her information' (Freud 1935a).[5]

Freud was biased against the daughter due to his opinion of the mother. He believed almost everything she told him. For decades Fanny Moser senior manipulated the people surrounding her, especially her various doctors, including Freud. At the time he agreed to come to Au in order to give his opinion on her daughter, Freud was 'instrumentalised' by her, and did not realise that he was a victim of her manipulations.

In conclusion, Freud was well aware of the shortcomings of his therapeutic technique in the late 1880s and early 1890s. He realised that he lacked experience in interpreting patients' accounts of situations and relationships. However, Freud is not famous for readily admitting his errors. His letters to Fanny Moser's daughter, then, are important documents, with respect to Freud's biography, and to the history of psychoanalysis.

Notes

1 See Andersson 1979: 7, 1960, 1962a.

2 'Ich kann es Ihnen nicht übel nehmen, daß Sie meinen schlimmen diagnostischen Irrtum von damals noch nicht verziehen haben. Nicht nur daß ich noch sehr unerfahren war, unser aller Kunst das seelisch Verborgene zu lesen, war noch in den Kinderschuhen. Zehn, vielleicht fünf Jahre später, hätte ich nicht umhin können zu erraten, daß die unglückliche Frau einen schweren Kampf gegen die unbew. Haß regungen für ihre beiden Kinder führte und sich durch überzärtlichkeit zu verteidigen suchte. Diese bösen Geister scheinen sich später zur Oberfläche durchgearbeitet und ihre Handlungen bestimmt zu haben. Aber damals verstand ich nichts u glaubte einfach ihrer Information.'

3 There is another letter from Freud to Fanny Moser junior from 1918, partly published by Andersson (1977), in which Freud again admits his mistaken diagnosis.

4 'Von Ihrem Buch habe ich mehrere Abschnitte gelesen. Ich anerkenne es als eine tapfere und ehrliche That, einen Schritt auf dem steinigsten Arbeitspfad. Daß ich die rein theoret. Kapitel Hypnot, Traum, Hysterie, besonders aber über das "Unterbew." nicht ganz gutheißen kann, wird Sie nicht verwundern.'

5 'Aber damals verstand ich nichts und glaubte einfach ihrer Information.'

FREUD'S NEURAL UNCONSCIOUS

David L. Smith

Introduction

In this paper I will examine aspects of the evolution of Freud's philosophy of mind. In particular, I will investigate his views on the 'mind-body problem' and the concept of unconscious mental events.

Notions of 'the unconscious' were widespread in the second half of the nineteenth century (Ellenberger 1970; Whyte 1978). It is less frequently noted that these concepts were far from homogeneous. Several distinct ideas of the unconscious were advocated by philosophers, psychologists and neuroscientists during that period. In order to understand these notions, and Freud's relationship to them, it is essential to grasp the fact that they were, on the whole, nested within a dualistic philosophical framework.

Descartes formalised a sophisticated *interactionist* theory of the mind-body relationship in the seventeenth century. According to this theory, the immaterial mind interacts with the material body through the medium of the pineal gland. The main difficulty of this thesis became apparent almost immediately. How can a material substance interact with an immaterial substance? At what common point can they meet? The theory of *psycho-physical parallelism* arose as a response to this problem. According to this view, mental and physical events did not interact at all; they were merely co-ordinated with one another. In order to make this 'pre-established harmony' plausible, many felt it necessary to invoke God as its architect.

Scientific developments occurring around the middle of the nineteenth century made traditional forms of dualism increasingly difficult to sustain. Amongst these were: Mayer's discovery of the law of the conservation of energy, which refuted interactionism[1]; Darwin's theory of evolution, which suggested that mental faculties have evolved in response to physical selection pressures; and the developing field of neuroscience, which demonstrated the causal dependence of mental capacities upon neurophysiological processes.[2]

A significant and widely advocated response to the challenge posed by these developments was the theory of *epiphenomenalism*. Epiphenomenalists proposed that the brain possesses non-physical properties that are, however, devoid of causal powers. The wetware of the brain determines what goes on in the mind. The mind can influence neither neurophysiological nor mental processes. It should be borne in mind that epiphenomenalism remained within the purview of dualism. Epiphenomenalists did not take the final step to materialism by *equating* mind and brain. In the absence of concepts of artificial intelligence, such a step must have seemed wildly counter-intuitive to all but the most adventurous thinkers.

Theories of the unconscious

To return to nineteenth century theories of the unconscious, there seem to have been at least three prevalent views. Some philosophers treated the unconscious in mystical and universalistic terms, in accord with the metaphysical extravagance of German-language philosophy during this period. The most influential proponent of this approach was probably Edouard von Hartmann, who wrote—in his celebrated *Philosophy of the Unconscious*—that we 'merge into an eternal Unconscious, into a unique, omnipresent, and omniscient all-wise being' (Brentano 1973a: 108). Others, working within parallelist and epiphenomenalist frameworks, claimed that so-called unconscious mental events were really just neurophysiological *dispositions* for (by definition, conscious) mental events. According to this view, unconscious events are not mental at all. Gustav Fechner, who was read and admired by Freud, wrote that:

> Sensations, ideas, have, of course, *ceased actually* to exist in the state of unconsciousness, insofar as we consider them apart from their substructure. Nevertheless something persists within us, ie. the psychophysical activity of which they are a function, and which makes possible the reappearance of sensation, etc. (Brentano 1973a: 104)

The dispositionalist approach was also endorsed by Franz Brentano and John Hughlings Jackson, both of whom exerted a powerful influence on Freud's intellectual development.

A third view, advocated mainly by French writers, argued that so-called unconscious states should be explained in terms of the splitting or 'doubling' (*'doublement'*) of *consciousness*. These theorists, who included Taine, Dessoir, Binet, Paul and Pierre Janet, claimed that unconscious states were not intrinsically unconscious, but were analogous to conscious states in other minds. The split-consciousness theory was closely, although by no means exclusively, associated with attempts to explain the dynamics of hysteria and the phenomenon of post-hypnotic suggestion.

Of course, scientific investigators were inclined to eschew the mystical notion of the unconscious in favour of one of the others.[3] Flournoy (1995) regarded the dispositional and split-consciousness views as the main contenders and as mutually exclusive.

> The words *subliminal* (*sub limen, unter der schwelle*, under the threshold), and *subconscious* or *unconscious* are practically synonymous and designate phenomena and processes that one has some reason to believe are conscious even though they are unknown to the subject, since they take place so to speak below the level of its ordinary consciousness. The question, of course, remains open to knowledge, if and up to what point, in each particular case, these hidden processes are really accompanied by consciousness, or whether they go back to the pure mechanism of 'unconscious cerebration',[4] in which case the expression 'subliminal consciousness' can no longer be applied but metaphorically, which is, however, no reason to banish it. (Flournoy 1995: 8)

This passage illustrates the deep-rootedness and dire consequences of dualist intuitions for nineteenth century psychology. It is important to bear in mind that *introspectionism* was also part of the Cartesian psychological heritage. Descartes held that the mind is transparent and incorrigible with respect to its own contents. It followed that psychological research should be conducted by means of introspection, by studying the revealed content of one's own mind. The period that Lyons (1986) has called the 'golden age of introspection' lasted from the seventeenth right up to the beginning of the twentieth century.

Of course, the very notion of unconscious mental events posed a challenge to the introspectionist program, for an unconscious event is by definition outside the scope of our introspective capacities. Both dispositionalist and split-consciousness theories were, however, able to preserve introspectionist intuitions in the face of apparently recalcitrant data. The dispositionalist could accept the existence of unconscious events whilst *denying* that these possessed a truly mental character. The split-consciousness theorist could claim that the sub-personality giving rise to ostensibly 'unconscious' states has Cartesian access to its own mental states, notwithstanding the fact that these states are unintrospectable by the subject's 'main' consciousness. According to this view we are unconscious of our own mental contents in just the same way that we are unconscious of other people's mental states.[5]

Freud's dualistic and pre-topographical phase

Prior to 1895, Freud, in common with most of his colleagues, worked within the dualist tradition. His article 'Gehirn' (Freud 1990) is clearly dualistic, as is his paper on 'Psychical (or Mental) Treatment' (Freud 1890). In *On Aphasia* (Freud 1953) Freud explicitly endorsed Jackson's (1887) 'doctrine of concomitance', a form of psychophysical parallelism. All of Freud's works written prior to April 1895 either endorse or are compatible with some form of dualism.[6]

Herzog (1991) has noted that none of Freud's pre-1896 writings make use of the concept of a mental unconscious. At some points Freud deployed the dispositionalist theory and at other times he advocated the split-consciousness theory. An example of the former can be found in 'The Neuro-Psychoses of Defence' (1894). The latter is particularly marked in the *Studies on Hysteria* (Breuer & Freud 1895).[7]

Herzog demonstrates that Freud's use of the concept of a mental unconscious made its public debut in the three papers on the seduction theory published in the spring of 1896. Of course, it is impossible to know with certainty just what led Freud to change his views at this time, but there are hints in his writings which provide a basis for some inferences. To my mind, the following passage from Freud's chapter on the psychotherapy of hysteria in the *Studies on Hysteria* is crucial in this connection.

> The ideas which are derived from the greatest depth and which for the nucleus of the pathogenic organisation are also those which are acknowledged as memories by the patient with the greatest difficulty. Even when everything is finished and the patients have been overborne by the force of logic and have been convinced by the therapeutic effect accompanying the emergence of precisely these ideas—when, I say, the patients themselves accept the fact that they thought this or that, they often add: 'But I can't *remember* having thought it'. It is easy to come to

> terms with them by telling them that the thoughts were *unconscious*. But how is this state of affairs to be fitted into our own psychological views? (Breuer & Freud 1895: 300)

Freud's problem here was how to explain the fact that his patients were unable to identify his inferences about their pathogenic memories as accounts of their own *experiences*, even in cases where the communication of these inferences produced some therapeutic effect. Freud continued:

> Are we to disregard this withholding of recognition on the part of patients, when, now that the work is finished, there is no longer any motive for their doing so? Or are we to suppose that we are really dealing with thoughts which never came about, which merely had a *possibility* of existing, so that the treatment would lie in the accomplishment of a psychical act which did not take place at the time? (Breuer & Freud 1895: 300)

The implications of these comments can only be appreciated in light of the split-consciousness and dispositionalist theories. Recall that Freud and Breuer based the *Studies* on a split-consciousness model of hysteria. According to this model, in order to eliminate hysterical symptoms it is only necessary to restore integrity to a previously divided consciousness through inducing hysterical patients to accept the (inferred) pathogenic ideas believed to form the nucleus of the dissociated portion of consciousness. Freud's patients did not feel that his inferences corresponded to their *experiences*,[8] a result that was inconsistent with the split-consciousness model.

In the passage reproduced above, Freud went on to consider the possibility that so called unconscious or dissociated contents may just be neurophysiological dispositions. Therapy is reconceptualised in terms of realising latent dispositions rather than restoring unity to the self. Unwilling to commit himself to this alternative, Freud continued:

> It is clearly impossible to say anything about this—that is, about the state which the pathogenic material was in before the analysis—until we have arrived at a thorough clarification of our basic psychological views, especially on the nature of consciousness. (Breuer & Freud 1895: 300)

Freud's transition to materialism and the mental unconscious

This undertaking was launched less than a month later in the form of what is now called the 'A Project for a Scientific Psychology'.[9] The 'Project' was initiated with the intention of explaining 'defence'—that is, explaining how a mental content can be excluded from consciousness—by means of an elaborate physicalistic model of the mind providing the 'thorough clarification' promised in the *Studies*.[10] Philosophically speaking, the great achievement of the 'Project' was the transition from dualism to a version of the identity theory: the thesis that mental states are brain states. Freud announced his new-found materialism at the beginning of the 'Project':

> The intention is to furnish a psychology that shall be a natural science: that is, to represent psychical processes as quantitatively determinate states of specifiable material particles, thus making those processes perspicuous and free from contradiction. (Freud 1950: 295)

As is well known, the 'Project' attempted to explain mental processes in terms of three hypothetical neural systems: the φ neurones, ψ neurones and ω neurones. The φ neurones constitute the input (sensory) channels of the 'apparatus', the ψ neurones make up the representation-generating system, the home of mental 'content', while the ω neurones make up the consciousness-producing system. In separating intentionality (a property of ψ) from consciousness (a property of ω), Freud made room for a *physicalistic* concept of unconscious mental events. He was quick to appreciate the anti-Cartesian epistemological implications of his new ontology. If, as Freud claimed, the becoming conscious of a mental content is just φ causing an effect in ω, then consciousness is no longer regarded as having unmediated access to its own contents and processes.

> We at once become clear about a postulate which has been guiding us up to now. We have been treating psychical processes as something that could dispense with this awareness through consciousness, as something that exists independently of this awareness. We are prepared to find that some of our assumptions are not confirmed through consciousness, as something that exists independently of such awareness. If we do not let ourselves be

> confused on that account, it follows, from the postulate of consciousness providing neither complete nor trustworthy knowledge of the neuronal processes, that these are in the first instance to be regarded to their whole extent as unconscious and are to be inferred like other natural things. (Freud 1950: 308)

This is a far cry from earlier claims that mental events can be characterised only introspectively and non-physicalistically (for example, Freud 1990). By the spring of 1896 Freud had come to believe not only that consciousness cannot intuitively grasp its own basis but also that mental states can, in principle, be given purely neurophysiological specifications.

I have already mentioned what appears to have been Freud's main clinical reason for rejecting the split consciousness theory.[11] An alternative response to the apparent falsification of the deductive consequences of this theory would have been for Freud to retain his belief in the theory whilst regarding his cures as placebo effects. With regard to the dispositionalist theory, there were obvious clinical grounds for its rejection. According to Freud's clinical theory, neurotic symptoms are sustained by intrapsychic conflict. It is difficult to imagine how a mental state could enter into conflict with or indeed enter into any logical relation with a non-mental neurophysiological disposition. Freud's theory of intrapsychic conflict describes conflict between states that are both occurrent and mental.[12]

Later, Freud (1915b, 1926, 1940) used a rather different argument to neutralise the dispositionalist thesis. I have christened this the 'continuity argument'.[13] Here is how he put it in 'The Unconscious':

> The data of consciousness have a very large number of gaps in them; both in healthy and in sick people psychical acts often occur which can be explained only by presupposing other acts, of which, nevertheless, consciousness affords no evidence... Our most personal daily experience acquaints us with ideas that come into our head, we do not know from where, and with intellectual conclusions arrived at we do not know how. (Freud 1915b: 166-167)

The strongest case of gaps in consciousness implying unconscious mental work is the example of a seemingly intractable intellectual problem which, after having been consciously abandoned at time T^1

issues in a solution suddenly occurring to one at T^2 without the benefit of any conscious work being done on the problem during the interval between T^1 and T^2 'as is shown when someone finds, immediately after waking, that he knows the solution to a difficult mathematical problem with which he had been wrestling in vain the day before' (Freud 1923: 26).[14] According to the dispositionalist thesis, there was no mental work on the problem during the period between T^1 and T^2, but this is clearly implausible. If we grant that neurophysiological processes secure the continuity between the vents at T^1 and T^2 we must also grant that these neurophysiological processes are mental as well.

Conclusion

1895 was a watershed for Freud. It was the year in which he exchanged his conventional dualism for a more audacious espousal of the identity theory.[15] It was the year that he embraced a full-blooded conception of intrinsically unconscious mental events nested within his materialist theory of mind. Arguably, it was the year that he invented psychoanalysis, the 'science of the mental unconscious' (Freud 1926: 231). Freud unswervingly affirmed his concept of the neural unconscious for the remainder of his life.[16]

Freud's criticism of the philosophical systems of his day centred on their rationalism and their anti-naturalism. Now, in the 1990s, philosophers and cognitive scientists routinely advocate materialist conceptions of mind. Freud's complaint that philosophers axiomatically equate mental with conscious mental events is no longer widely applicable. In this respect, Freud emerges as an strikingly contemporary thinker. As Robert Solomon has stated:

> Freud is often criticised for his philosophical naivety, largely on the basis of his 'confusing' mentalistic and biological categories and remaining ignorant of the complexities of psychophysical dualism... Freud was not only aware of these problems, but was one of the very few psychologists or philosophers of his time (the other being William James) who began to see the serious problems in the linguistic and metaphysical conservatism that provided the inertia of Cartesian dualism in psychology. (Solomon 1987: 138)

Notes

[1] See, for example, Jackson 1887, who described the belief that mental items cause physical events as implying disbelief in the law of the conservation of energy. 'Movements', he wrote, 'always arise from liberations of energy in the outer world, and it would be marvellous if there were an exception in our brains...' (Jackson 1887: 86). Jackson's own commitment to psychophysical parallelism was, however, scarcely more plausible. As William James remarked 'this "concomitance" in the midst of "absolute separateness" is an utterly irrational notion' (James 1950: 136).

[2] Many nineteenth-century neuroscientists nevertheless retained a belief in the traditional forms of dualism. Fritsch, Hitzig and Flourens were Cartesian interactionists, while Jackson and Ferrier were psychophysical parallelists (Young 1970).

[3] Dalbiez (1941) seems to be the only writer clearly to distinguish Freud's philosophical conception of the unconscious from its rivals, and to distinguish the two main rivals from one another. He describes Freud's concept as a 'realist' view in that it distinguishes mental events from our perceptions of those events. He describes the rival views as 'idealist' in that they fail to draw this distinction. Dalbiez describes the two main idealist views as the 'physiological theory' (my 'dispositional theory') and the 'theory of the plurality of centres of consciousness' (my 'split consciousness theory').

[4] This term was introduced by Carpenter (1874).

[5] Donald Davidson's (1982) philosophical reconstruction of Freud's theory of the unconscious (mis)interprets it as a version of the split consciousness theory. Searle (1992) criticises Freud's theory using the dispositionalist theory. Both of these authors seem ignorant of the philosophical disputes about the unconscious during Freud's lifetime and of the fact that Freud explicitly rejected both split consciousness and dispositionalist theories on good philosophical grounds.

[6] I do not know whether this holds true in relation to Freud's untranslated works.

[7] See also Freud's (1893) lecture 'On the Psychical Mechanism of Hysterical Phenomena', where he claims that: 'it is probable that in every hysteria we are dealing with a rudiment of what is called [in French] "*double conscience*", dual consciousness, and that a tendency to such a dissociation and with it the emergence of abnormal states of consciousness... is the basic phenomenon of hysteria' (Freud 1893e: 38-39).

[8] A good example is Illona Weiss, the subject of Freud's celebrated case of Elisabeth von R. in the *Studies*, who described Freud to her daughter as having tried to persuade her that she was in love with her brother in law 'but that wasn't really so' (Gay 1988: 72).

[9] The 'Project' is first mentioned explicitly in a letter to Fliess dated 27th April, 1895. However, the letter implies that Freud had previously mentioned this research to his friend, perhaps on the occasion of one of their 'congresses'. It is clear that Freud began working on the 'Project' some time after 4th March, because in the letter bearing that date, Freud mentions that he is not up to much scientific work apart from hurriedly writing the chapter on psychotherapy for the *Studies*. The letter of 8th March states much the same. On the 13th he mentions having completed fifty-two pages of the chapter, and having an 'inkling of new ideas' (Masson 1985: 120). On 28th March he describes being 'plagued' by psychology but devoid of ideas. On 11th April he states that he has worked himself 'to the bone' on psychology. I reconstruct from these facts that Freud wrote the passages from *Studies on Hysteria* dealing with the problem of the unconscious around the middle of March. He was preoccupied with the issues raised, but had no idea of how to deal with them until some time around the beginning of April, when the 'Project' was apparently initiated.

[10] Freud wrote to Fliess on 16 August that: 'All I was trying to do was explain defence... I had to work my way through the problem of quality, sleep, memory—in short, all of psychology' (Masson 1985: 136).

[11] Twenty years later in 'The Unconscious' (1915b) Freud raised additional philosophical objections to the split-consciousness theory.

[12] I am not aware of any place in his writings where Freud raises these issues.

[13] It seems, likely that Freud took the continuity argument from the Scottish philosopher Sir William Hamilton. We know that Freud was acquainted with Mill's (1865) critique of Hamilton from a footnote to *On Aphasia* (Freud 1953, first published 1891). Mill's chapter fifteen is entitled 'Sir William Hamilton's Doctrine of Unconscious Mental Modifications'. Mill cites Hamilton (1853), who stated that: 'It sometimes happens, that we find one thought rising immediately after another in consciousness, but whose consecution we can reduce to no law of association. Now in these cases we can generally discover by an attentive observation, that these two thoughts, though not themselves associated, are each associated with certain other thoughts, so that the whole consecution would have been regular, had these intermediate thoughts come into consciousness, between the two which are not immediately associated' (Mill 1865: 352-353). Mill attempts to refute Hamilton, first by claiming that conscious links between the associations have simply been forgotten and then by invoking a version of the dispositional argument: 'It may well be believed that the apparently suppressed links in a chain of association, those which Sir W. Hamilton considers as latent, really are so; the chain of causation being continued only physically, by one organic state of the nerves succeeding another so rapidly that the state of mental consciousness appropriate to each is not produced' (Mill 1865: 282-283).

[14] There are marvellous examples of this process in Hadamard (1949) and Koestler (1964).

[15] I am of course aware that a number of scholars do not agree with me on the point. The major battle-positions are as follows. Andersson (1962b) claims that Freud was an epiphenomenalist. Silverstein (1985, 1989) describes him as an interactionist, Young (1970), Solms and Saling (1986, 1990) and Sulloway (1979) describe him as a parallelist. Holt (1974) states that Freud was inconsistent. Amongst those scholars with whom I am in substantial agreement on this issue are Amacher (1965), Natsoulas (1974), Solomon (1987), Flanagan (1986), Mackay (1989) and Wallace (1992).

[16] I am in agreement with Solomon (1987) who claims that Freud abandoned the 'Project' because of the limitations of the neuroscience of his day. This is consistent with Freud's remark at a meeting of the Vienna Psycho-Analytic Society on 20th October, 1909 that such problems 'may be on the agenda a century after us' (Nunberg & Federn, 1962-75: 280).

THE TOPOLOGY OF 'A PROJECT FOR A SCIENTIFIC PSYCHOLOGY'

Nathalie Charraud

Freud and Saussure

As Lacan pointed out on several occasions, Saussure's linguistic theory would have perfected Freud's theory of the unconscious, by complementing it with a theory of the signifier. In advancing the notion that the unconscious is structured like a language, Lacan was only making explicit what Freud himself had said.

What interests me in this is that these—let us say—linguistic foundations of the definition of the unconscious were already present in the 'A Project for a Scientific Psychology' (Freud 1950). In effect, Freud's 'quantities of energy' play a considerable role, when moving from one neuron to another, because these movements materialise associations between neurons which carry the inscription, or writing, of a representation.[1]

As far as I could judge from the French translation, the term representation [idea] only appears in the text in very precise contexts, when the clinical issues raised by the dream or the hysterical or obsessional symptom are under discussion. It is mainly in the second section of the 'Project'—entitled 'Psychopathology'—that the term 'representation' becomes useful. Indeed, it is indispensable for an explanation of hysterical phenomena: elements become pathogenic in cases of 'excessively intense ideas', when the charge becomes too strong. The term does not appear until the end of the first section, where Freud examines the dream of Irma's injection (Freud 1950: 341-2), to which he returns in *The Interpretation of Dreams* (1900). Oddly enough, the third section of the 'Project', which is concerned with normal processes of thought, departs once again from the notion of representation.

My opinion, then, is that it was the 'pathological' aspect of the dream and the symptom which prompted Freud to develop the notion of the unconscious in the way that he did, some years later.

Guy Trobas has raised the question of how we might identify the precise moment at which Freud invented psychoanalysis. He rightly suggested that the answer is to be found in 'the primary and fundamental concept of psychoanalysis, namely the unconscious' (Trobas

1999). Freud himself marked this inaugural moment, when he fully interpreted the dream of Irma's injection, by imagining a marble plaque commemorating the event (Masson 1985: 417). In the 'Project', the paragraph devoted to Irma stands out and defines the science of psychoanalysis in opposition to psychology or physiology. This inaugural moment is what Lacan later described as S_1—S_2, the set of signifiers reduced to its simplest expression. The significance of this can be approached in several ways, one of which is the way that Freud interprets his own dream:

> C has taken the place of B, though B fits in better with the connection of thought, with the wish-fulfilment. (Freud 1950: 341)

If B does not appear immediately in Freud's associations, it is because of its *sexual* connotation.

It is here, then, that we witness the moment which—it seems to me—inaugurates psychoanalysis. Moreover Freud, who was a contemporary of Saussure, here comes very close to the great linguist, with this theory of representations, chains and associations. Additionally Freud, with the notion of 'purposive representation' (cf. Freud 1900: 528-31) introduced a specific orientation into the networks of signifiers—these representations have a sexual signification. Epistemologists and historians of science are better placed to say why, at the end of the nineteenth century, the time was ripe for the elaboration of a theory of the unconscious, and of a theory of language, both of which are related, as Lacan so brilliantly demonstrated.

A topology of signifiers

In his seminar on Ethics, Lacan invites us to re-read the 'Project' from a topological point of view. How might we respond to this invitation?

On a global level, the topology of the 'Project' presents us with a paradox. The system ϕ (perception), situated on the exterior, must—Freud proposes—somehow join the system ω (consciousness). However (and Lacan draws our attention to this oddity), system ψ is situated between perception and consciousness. This global topology of the subject will be elucidated by Lacan with the Moebius band or the projective plane (or cross-cap), which can account for how the most distal point can join the most proximal point. The torus can also solve this aporia.

On the other hand, a strictly local topology leads us to the signifier. A topology of the signifier is a topology which locates each signifier within a set of neighbourhoods—a key notion of general topology. The neighbourhood of a signifier corresponds to a group of other signifiers, which are in a relation of proximity to it.

The notion of the neighbourhood of the signifier is found in Saussure, under the heading of what he terms 'associative groupings'. He states:

> Outside the context of discourse, words having something in common are associated together in the memory. In this way they form groups, the members of which may be related in various ways. (Saussure 1983: 171)

In the 'Project', Freud refers not only to relations of association through chains or networks, but, through the notion of 'complex', refers in exactly the same way as Saussure to the notion of *multiple* forms of relationship between the elements:

> For the time has come to remember that perceptual cathexes are never cathexes of single neurons but always of complexes. (Freud 1950: 327)

Here, Freud is referring to the synchronic structure of signifiers, in which Lacan locates the mechanisms of the primary processes. The diachronic development of speech, on the other hand, implies the syntagmatic string of the secondary process.

We can make the topological character of the notion of neighbourhood even clearer by opposing it to a geometric spatialisation. For Saussure, the associative groupings are formed neither in a definite number nor in a determined order—that is to say, they represent open sets and their elements are not spatially ordered. To talk about them, we must invoke a structure other than Euclidian geometry. This intuition is not shared by Freud, since the neuronic support requires a repartition in space. However, the way in which Lacan adopts the mechanisms of displacement and condensation, by making them equivalent to metonymy and metaphor respectively, can easily be described in topological terms.[2]

I would like to return here to a subtle topological notion that we find in both Freud and Saussure, but expressed in different terms—the notion of separation. For Saussure, signification depends on difference, on the opposition of a signifier to all the other signifiers which are in proximity to it. For there to be signification, each signifier must then be located at the centre of a constellation, 'from which connected terms radiate ad infinitum' (Saussure 1983: 174). It is therefore not sufficient simply for the topology of neighbourhoods to obtain; the signifier must also distinguish itself from any neighbouring signifier. In topological terms, it is said that the topology must be separated. If $S_1 \neq S_2$, then there exist two neighbourhoods, S_1 and S_2, which do not overlap—that is, whose intersection is empty. The separation of the topology results in there being no perfect synonyms—something with which most linguists will agree.

The clinical dimension of the 'Project'

How can this topological notion of separation be transposed into Freud's 'paths of conduction'? In fact, this very notion is already present in the 'Project'.

A complex is defined by the associative relations between the signifiers—that is, by *fixed* paths between the corresponding neurons. It is vital to understand what is meant by the 'fixity' of fixed paths in order to understand 'pathology', such as Freud describes it in the 'Project'. On the subject of hysterical repression he writes:

> it is symbol-formation of this stable kind which is the function that goes beyond normal defence. (Freud 1950: 352).

If the *fixed* paths are indispensable for associative relations, and thus for the humus of thought, nevertheless they become pathogenic and a source of symptoms if they are *immutable*.

Normality can thus be described as follows: even though there is a fixed path between S and S′, this must not be immutable. In terms of the topology of signifiers, this means precisely that S and S′ must be *separable*. The topological notion of separation thus permits one to introduce a distinction between neighbouring signifiers ('fixed paths') and non-separated signifiers ('immutable paths'). Without this, the clinical dimension of the 'Project' would remain somewhat obscure.

In fact, Freud says that the difficulty, the key to the problem, lies in the mechanism of repression. He indicates two different kinds of repression. The first kind corresponds to hysteria and depends on 'symbolisation'—that is, the non-separated link between a repressed element and an element which represents it. The second kind, which is found in obsessional neurosis, is a repression without symbolisation, a repression of a signifier in which all the signifier's associative paths have been blocked. Such a signifier, separated from all others, can be called *isolated*. This second type of repression is correlated to a too radical 'separation'. Thus, both non-separation and a separation which is too radical—due to the lack of neighbourhoods—are causes of neurotic symptoms.

Notes

1 *Vorstellung* is translated as 'idea' in the English translation, but here we prefer *'representation'*.

2 I have discussed this elsewhere. See Charraud 1997.

THE SYMPTOM AS METAPHOR: FREUD'S 'PROJECT'

Rivka Warshawsky

Scientifically, I am in a bad way; namely, caught up in 'The Psychology for Neurologists', which regularly consumes me totally until, actually overworked, I must break off. I have never before experienced such a high degree of preoccupation. (Masson 1985: letter from Freud to Fliess, 27th April, 1895)

...a man like me cannot live without a hobbyhorse, without a consuming passion, without—in Schiller's words—a tyrant. I have found one. In its service I know no limits. It is psychology... I am tormented by two aims: to examine what shape the theory of mental functioning takes if one introduces quantitative considerations, a sort of economics of nerve forces, and, second, to peel off from psychopathology a gain for normal psychology. (Masson 1985: letter dated 25th May, 1895)

Reporting on it now would be like sending a six-month foetus of a girl to a ball. (Masson 1985: letter dated 12th June, 1895)

I hope it is not 'dream gold'. (Masson 1985: letter dated 6th August, 1895)

...new difficulties... I threw the whole thing aside and am persuading myself that I am not in the least bit interested in it. It makes me quite uncomfortable to think that I am supposed to tell you about it. (Masson 1985: letter dated 16th August, 1895)

...in the process [I] became alternately proud and overjoyed and ashamed and miserable—until now, after an excess of mental torment, I apathetically tell myself: it does not yet, perhaps never will, hang together. (Masson 1985: letter dated 8th October, 1895)

Everything seemed to fall into place, the cogs meshed, I had the impression that the thing now really was a machine that shortly would function on its own... Naturally, I can scarcely manage to

> contain my delight. (Masson 1985: letter dated 20th October, 1895)

> I have packed up the psychological manuscripts, and thrown them into a drawer... incapable of mastering it all. (Masson 1985: letter dated 8th November, 1895)

Introduction

In November 1895, Freud wrote to Fliess concerning the 'Project for a Scientific Psychology':

> I no longer understand the state of mind in which I hatched the psychology; cannot conceive how I could have inflicted it on you. I believe you are still too polite; to me it appears to have been a kind of madness. (Masson 1985: 152)

The correspondence with Fliess indeed bears evidence of 'a kind of madness' where the 'Project' is concerned—or, at least, several extreme mood swings. However, one cannot overlook the fact that, at that time, Freud's 'state of mind' was directly influenced by the terrible 'Emma Eckstein incident'. The 'Project' was conceived just as Emma Eckstein appeared to be finally recovering from what can only be described as a serious mistake on the part of Fliess, who left some surgical gauze in her nose after operating on her.

Fliess' negligence in Emma Eckstein's case, her subsequent suffering and bleeding, together with the actual danger to her life, were clearly very traumatic for Freud, who was deeply affected and depressed. However, Freud went to great lengths to avoid attributing any blame or responsibility to his sensitive friend, who had operated on Freud himself at the very same time. Freud even went so far as to apologise to Fliess, for involving him in this distressing case!

Freud refrained from inflicting any hint of malpractice on Fliess, and instead—it seems—he inflicted the 'Project' on himself. Out of Freud's inability to admit to himself the flaw he had found in Fliess (the flaw in the Other) this symptomatic work—'a six-month foetus going to a ball'—was born, perhaps prematurely. Freud could not afford to face this harsh truth just then, and so he had to cover up its devastating effects upon him somehow. His genius certainly more than compensated for this incident, by producing the astonishing 'Project'.

We know that soon after this point the 'Project' was abandoned by Freud in disgust, and only resurfaced on its posthumous publication. It has been described as 'an abortive work' (Forrester 1980: 38), but is by no means a still-birth. Freud re-worked the structure and ideas of the 'Project' many times in his later works—consider, for example, chapter seven of *The Interpretation of Dreams* (Freud 1900) and *An Outline of Psycho-Analysis* (Freud 1940). Furthermore, the symbolic integration of the 'Project' into psychoanalytic history has been an ongoing process ever since its publication.

The formerly disregarded text of the 'Project' has thus acquired a unique value—it is a strange piece of rejected history, which, nevertheless, has not been obliterated or lost. The density of the theoretical work which it comprises is truly astonishing:

> ...the 'Project' stands as the greatest effort Freud ever made to force a mass of psychical facts within the framework of a quantitative theory, and as the demonstration by way of the absurd that the content exceeds the frame: not even in Chapter Seven of the *Traumdeutung* will Freud try to make so many things fit together within such a narrow system. (Ricoeur 1970: 73)

These properties of the 'Project'—its resurrection, its theoretical density—provide the most fruitful material for integrative reworking.

Reading Freud

The special work that the 'Project' has caused is, nevertheless, very similar to the kind of work that all Freud's texts require—namely the kind of 'reading' that Jacques Lacan instilled so well, and which is, in itself, a characteristically 'psychoanalytic' reading.

There exists a retroactive interplay between later texts and earlier ones, an articulation which consists in a reworking of the concepts and the resulting problems. In order to discover this articulation, one must trace the modifications in Freud's ideas. What problems in the 'Project' led to a different treatment of ensuing ideas and models? What went 'wrong': what did not mesh, or was lacking or excessive in the 'Project'? What problems arose from the endeavour to conceive of the entire psyche in the form embraced by the 'Project'? This form partly resembles a modern day mathematical axiomatic system; starting from two axiomatic principles, and one basic binary distinction (between 'cathected' and 'discharged' states), Freud endeavoured to prove a series of propositions which would account for the entire functioning of the psyche, without having recourse to biological explanations or to metapsychology. (Later, Lacan interpolated the order of the *real* in the place of what Freud called 'the recourse to biological explanations'.)

This kind of reading and retrospective reworking is described by Freud himself when he addressed the structure of the hysterical symptom in the second section of the 'Project', which deals with psychopathology. Here, Freud describes the hysterical 'Proton Pseudos'. This is a Greek term taken from Aristotle's *Prior Analytics* which means 'a false conclusion by way of a false premise'. We will see that the hysterical Proton Pseudos is based on a model of trauma, which will guide us directly towards the metaphoric structure of the symptom (that is, the linguistic connection of psychoanalysis). Secondly, the Proton Pseudos will lead us to the analytic interpretation as something touching on the real (that is, the *scientific* connection of psychoanalysis) and, thirdly, it will take us from the Cartesian methodology to the psychoanalytic discourse itself (the point at which psychoanalysis becomes *unique*, and separates itself from both linguistics and science).

The link with the real is the key problem addressed by Freud in the 'Project', as can be demonstrated by an examination of his work on the symptom. Thus we will firstly address the connection scientific connection of psychoanalysis, before proceeding to examine the symptom as a metaphor.

Science and truth

Although psychoanalysis maintains a tie with science, it also diverges in an important way from the aims of science. Science aims to produce knowledge blindly, whereas psychoanalysis aims to produce truth blindly.

The function of truth can be illuminated by the character of Tiresias, who is the blind seer in Sophocles' *Oedipus Rex* (Soler 1996). Another way in which the classics can help us distinguish between scientific and psychoanalytic discourse is through the example of Socratic questioning, as presented in Plato's *Dialogues*. Socratic dialectical questioning has often been compared with psychoanalytic work. However, when Socrates subverts prejudice and existing knowledge by asking everyone he encounters the most unsettling and irritating questions, he is actually closer—in one important respect—to scientific discourse than to psychoanalysis. For example, when Socrates says to Meno: 'I am sorry, my dear Meno, not only do I not know whether "virtu" can be taught or not, I actually do not even clearly know what this "virtu" of yours is at all. Could you be so kind as to tell me what you mean by it?', he is looking for *absolute* knowledge, in the sense of an 'essence', an 'ideal'. Absolute knowledge is that upon which we can all agree, which leads to a consensus. Therefore Socrates, like science, is veering towards a Universal Ideal.

Freud, on the other hand, may well ask the same question and also subvert existing knowledge, but he does so with a very different aim. He is striving to obtain, not the essence or ideal, but rather the most different, singular, and particular point concerning *the subject*. Freud is thus conducting the subject away from the universal, towards the most idiosyncratic meaning his words have for him (Miller 1987).

So what we have in the case of psychoanalysis is a science of the *particular*, of the idiosyncrasy of the subject and the unconscious—but not the 'collective', Jungian unconscious. Although this idiosyncrasy of the Freudian subject is closer to total nonsense than to sense, it is not just any old nonsense, but a very precise and logical form of nonsense; an 'Alice-in-Wonderland' nonsense.

A crucial question is, however, the following: in this age of the scientific discourse, in this era of the great law of profit, what profit can possibly be derived for the universal pool of knowledge from a singular, never-to-be-repeated subject's truth? (Soler 1996: 61-2) In other words, if psychoanalysis is research, then what *kind* of research is it?

I will demonstrate this fundamentally Freudian way of questioning the subject's idiosyncratic nonsense by a very simple example, which will lead me back to the 'Project'. It is the example of another Emma (not Emma Eckstein) whose symptom is taken by Freud as a prototypical example in the 'Project'. Emma was afraid to go into shops alone, because she was worried that the shopkeepers would laugh at her clothes. She explained this fear by a memory from the age of twelve (that is, after puberty): she had entered a shop and had been frightened away by two shopkeepers who laughed at her clothes, one of whom she found sexually attractive.[1]

In Freud's view, not every neurotic fear or phenomenon comprises a symptom. Only under certain conditions will he classify something as a symptom. According to Freud, in the 'Project', a symptom must comprise two elements:-

- an excessively intense idea;
- a substitution: Idea A takes the place of Idea B.

In addition, a symptom has a core of non-sense; it is: '(a) unintelligible (b) incapable of being resolved by the activity of thought (c) incongruous in its structure' (Freud 1950: 348).

Once these conditions are fulfilled 'a pathological symbol formation' (Freud 1950: 348) takes place. This is different from a normal symbol in that the original idea (Idea B) is *repressed*, because it generates anxiety. In a normal case, on the other hand, the idea which the symbol represents is not repressed—'the knight *knows* the glove he adores, obtains its value from the lady's person'. For the neurotic, however, the *glove itself* seems to acquire the actual value, without the lady's person being involved. To quote Freud: 'The symbol has taken the place of the thing entirely' (Freud 1950: 349).

Symptom as metaphor

Lacan proposed that this substitution constitutes a linguistic metaphor (Lacan 1991). Furthermore, this kind of substitution is conceivable only on the basis of the positional relations in a sentence. What is important in the Freudian symptom, is that the metaphor is placed in the position of the *subject*. Thus, the metaphor both represents the missing subject while at the same time exactly marking the place of the subject's absence. However, in the symptom, the point where the metaphor occurs—that is, where the second signifier (S_2) comes into effect—represents something (S_1) which is not only absent now, but which was absent from the outset. This causes an unexpected structural 'twist', which prevents the symptom (structured as metaphor) from being a direct sign. A sign represents something to somebody—for example, for a physician a medical symptom is a sign of a certain referent or malady. The psychoanalytic symptom, however, does not represent a certain referent for anybody—not even for the individual bearing the symptom. This is because the subject is not the individual.

It immediately becomes obvious from the way in which Freud constructed his model of trauma, that a symptom is not a sign (Clastres 1990). This structure (of *Nachträglichkeit*) is present in all of Freud's cases-histories, but is mentioned quite explicitly in the 'Project' (Freud 1950: 353-6). According to Freud, a trauma consists of two moments in time (Scene II and Scene I). First, there is an encounter which was radically 'missed'. Although this moment is chronologically prior to Scene I, Freud calls it Scene II because it appears later in the patient's narrative, and only as a consequence of the analytic reconstructive work. Later, Freud will designate it the 'Other Scene'. The 'Other Scene' is what the analyst listens to beyond the patient's conscious narrative. Therefore, it constitutes the first moment of Freud's scheme (S_1). For instance, in the case of Emma, in the 'Project', she had an 'explanatory' memory from the age of twelve, clearly traumatic, which explained her present-day shop phobia (S_1). However the analytic work produced an even earlier memory, something that happened in a shop when she was a little girl (S_2).

For Emma the trauma did not occur until the second point, where the second memory (S_2), took the place of the first memory and substituted it ('Idea A takes the place of Idea B'). Oddly enough, it is at this point—and not at the first point—that the symptom is formed and the trauma fully experienced. The symptom develops because there is something in common between the two points. Somewhere in between the two points of the symptom lies the unconscious for Freud and the subject for Lacan.

$$\frac{S_1 \rightarrow S_2}{S}$$

Interpretation

Interpreting involves relating the second point to the first. In addition, in order to obtain some structure one must define a certain set of elements. There must be an axiom of specification which will lead us out of the impasse of the 'All' or the 'Everything'—in our case, 'All the possible meanings'. Language is the 'All' and the psychoanalytic discourse is that which extracts a certain set of signifiers from this 'All', a basic set in the sense of catalogue or class. For the analyst the elements of this set will constitute a definite limit on the possible meanings of the symptom. This is the link with scientific praxis.

If we look at the symptom of Emma in the 'Project' we find a point at which Freud says: this is the material at our disposal: (clothes, shop assistants, laughing, sexual feeling). Within the brackets Freud places the key signifiers from the patient's discourse, the common denominators between Scene II and Scene I. These elements of the basic set form the interposition of the Other's discourse between the narrative of the patient and the attentive analyst. This collection parallels the extraction of scientific data during an experimental procedure.

The unthought memory—S_1

However, what is particularly enigmatic and interesting here is the status of the first point, which Lacan termed a '*missed* encounter'.

Both moments of the trauma are not immediate perceptions, but are only memories. With regard to the first traumatic scene, we have what Freud describes as 'the case of a memory arousing an effect (much later) which it did not arouse [at all when] experienced' (Freud 1950: 356). Freud continues: 'Now this case is typical of repression in hysteria. We invariably find that a memory is repressed which has only become traumatic [afterwards] by *deferred action*' (Freud 1950: 356). The Other Scene failed to be represented and so needs to be staged in reality by a sequel scene or action, by the substitution point which then becomes the false neurotic connection or the 'Proton Pseudos'. In this way, then, in the case of Emma, the first inaccessible memory of the shopkeeper who assaulted her sexually *through* her clothes (that is, the 'unthought' memory), was staged in an enigmatic way by the sequel scene at a much later age, when she went into a shop and the assistants laughed *at* her clothes, and by her resultant fear of going into a shop by herself.

If this staging is successful, a memory is created the status of which has *changed* since its original registration.

It is worth describing the strange ontology and twisted temporality of the first traumatic memory once more, since it lies at the very heart of psychoanalysis proper:

> What has to be given life? Not what once was, nor what never was, but simply what has not been realised, what could have been, had the moment not been missed. (Anonymous 1994: 3-4)

This *real*—the 'unrealised'—leaves the traumatic memory as a hole in discourse and experience, giving rise to the Lacanian pun '*troumatic*'. It will 'appear' through the signifying repetition of the 'enactment of the reality of the unconscious', via the unconscious desires which come to life like vampires as soon as they taste blood.

Later, Freud developed the idea of the ontological change in the status of the first memory, which he laid out for the first time in the 'Project': only something which has once been a conscious perception can again become conscious and anything arising from within that seeks to become conscious must try to transform itself into an external perception (Freud 1923: 13-25). This feat is accomplished by Emma through her symptom, which stages the earlier, unconscious scene and provides an external perception of it, thus bringing it into psychic 'existence'.

This fundamentally original conception of trauma was present in psychoanalysis from the start. However, in the 'Project', Freud mistakenly attributed it to sexual 'development', thus succumbing to a biological explanation (which he had originally tried to exclude).

This in itself is an instance of causation being 'missed'. Instead, a smooth homogenous rule or inductive law was produced by Freud. This smooth law of progression from asexual infancy to genital maturity (both later refuted, by Freud himself, as fairy-tales) was found instead to be perturbed by the partial object of the libido—that is, by infantile sexuality and the partial drives, in order for the pure desire as an enigmatic cause to emerge. But this development did not take place in the 'Project'. In this respect, the 'Project' can be compared with Moses, who led the way to the Promised Land but did not actually enter it. Moses died outside its border, thus redoubling his importance as a signifier in the history of the Israelites.

In my view, the unitary signifier (S_1)—the function of which was fulfilled, for Freud, by the 'Project'—had to be linked to knowledge (S_2). Freud's later texts elaborated upon the structure of the 'Project' and dealt in a metaphorical manner with the ideas it contained. That is to say, in a manner which shed new light and new meanings on each of the psychoanalytic problems which Freud encountered for the first time whilst conceiving the 'Project'.

The psychoanalytic discourse

In the years following his 'A Project for a Scientific Psychology', Freud gradually began to grapple with some strange and baffling phenomena in psychoanalysis.

The symptom was no longer docile; it began to manifest itself. It could no longer be cured even by the most precise interpretations. The symbolic order did not function automatically and smoothly, and the 'holes' of the trauma became more and more apparent. Knowledge did not know, any longer, how to effect a cure. There was evidence of negative therapeutic reaction, the repetition compulsion, unconscious guilt, and a 'beyond' of the pleasure principle.

Something evidently remained outside of language, and psychoanalysis needed a way to grasp this something other than by interpreting the symptom. Freud turned more and more to 'reconstructions', and the linking of the symptom with fantasy. Language did not suffice, so the concept of a discourse imposed itself. The purpose of the discourse of psychoanalysis is to grasp what has been lost forever in language. This discourse is not a method, but a particular strategy to apprehend what has already escaped the method of language—a kind of 'quantity' or 'force' (which evokes the concept of 'Q' of the 'Project'). This discourse which is not a method cannot be replicated in tests of its reliability, but it can be written, it has its letters (Mauas 1989). It creates not an Aristotelian system of given categories into which the subjects being studied can be fitted, but a way in which each subject can, and should, produce a new category of absolute difference at the end of his analysis.

At one point in his composition of the 'Project', Freud wrote to Fliess that he had created a machine which would begin to run by itself at any moment. But, as with Descartes, Freud's efforts to impose a method on a given material served to reveal something which opposed the method, some real point of solidity at which the application broke. Ricoeur states that in the 'Project', Freud extended the scientific method of his time and 'transformed it to the breaking point'. In a similar manner, the constancy principle 'was transcended by its own applications' (Ricoeur 1970: 73).

Freud tried to build a post-Cartesian machine, freed from the burden of truth and lies; a symbolic grid which ran by itself, starting from first principles, and which referred to nothing outside itself. As in post-Cartesian science:

> Truth was set aside; it became a secondary consideration compared to that of applying to reality a symbolic grid, expressible in numeric terms, and developing the endless set of relations among the elements constituting that symbolic grid. (Fink 1995: 60)

The machine of knowledge is always brought to a standstill by the truths and half truths of hysteria which Freud, fortunately, never evaded. And the closed circuit of the constancy principle was broken at the point where the 'experience of satisfaction' introduced the Other, who would modify the autonomy of this circuit in a particular way for the subject. The 'Project for a Scientific Psychology' became Freud's life's work. John Forrester draws our attention to the astonishing similarity in layout and contents between the 'Project' and Freud's last expository work, *An Outline of Psycho-Analysis*. He also points out that the 'Mystic Writing Pad' (Freud 1925a) is Freud's last 'machine', and serves as an appendix to the 'Project' (Forrester 1980: 223).

Notes

[1] This symptom already makes us aware that the interpretative work should not necessarily be equated with an explanation. Emma already had a very clear explanation, but this did nothing to alleviate her symptom.

A READING OF AN ETHICS OF PSYCHOANALYSIS FROM FREUD'S FORMULATION OF *DAS DING* IN THE 'PROJECT FOR A SCIENTIFIC PSYCHOLOGY'

Helen Sheehan

Rilke asked in his letters, 'how is it possible to live when the fundamental of things, our life, is so incomprehensible,—when we are always inadequate in love, wavering in our determination and impotent in the face of death—how is it possible to exist?' (Rilke 1988: 264).

He continues: 'I have not managed to conquer my amazement at the fact that for thousands of years humanity has been concerning itself with life and death (not to speak of God) yet even today (and for how much longer?) stands in front of these primary—these immediate tasks (strictly speaking the only ones we have—for what else can we do?) So helplessly, so pitiably caught between terror and evasion like the veriest beginners. Is it not incredible? My amazement over this fact when I give way to it drives me into the greatest confusion and then into a sort of horror; but behind the horror there is something else; something so immediate and yet transcending all immediacy, something so intense that I cannot decide with my feeling whether it be like fire or ice' (Rilke 1988: 264).

The ethical dilemma laid bare before the apprehension of the horror—of the hostile Thing at the centre of existence—the psychoanalyst will deal with in a different way from the poet. What I hope to do here is to introduce the Freudian concept of *das Ding*—'the Thing'—as he outlined it in his 'A Project for a Scientific Psychology', a pre-analytical writing, which dates from 1895.

James Strachey, in his editor's introduction, says: 'what we have in the "Project" is a pre-id—a defensive description of the mind' (Strachey 1966: 292). My reading of the 'Project' and of *das Ding* in particular is that it is defensive after a manner and is couched in neurophysiological terms for two principal reasons. It seems to me to be the most intimate and revealing piece of work Freud ever engaged in, because it reveals his reflections on life and death and faith and love and forgiveness—it is in fact the trajectory of a psychoanalysis. No wonder, then, that Strachey says 'later in life he seems to have forgotten it or at least never to have referred to it' (Strachey 1966: 290). We can therefore stipulate that it was a successful analysis. The second thing that Freud seems to be saying in this 'Project' is how necessary it is to go via the body to engage with the Truth, because that way to the truth is the fact that *das Ding* is *the* fundamental Thing with which the human subject has to come to terms if he wishes to capture his little bit of space in the Real.

Das Ding is about many things—which I will try and elucidate as we proceed. However, Lacan says of it that it 'holds the secret'—and he is right. It certainly holds the key to desire and, in the Lacanian formulation, desire is the key to ethics.

The classical view of ethics is that one engages in ethical reflection in order to be moral. Freud's legacy is to highlight the precarious nature of that morality. Ethics, even as it reflects, could also fall into the trap of an ideal, and so if there is an ethics of psychoanalysis—and it is not clear from the outset that there is one—then one has to go the Freudian way to engage with that ethical dimension.

And that ethical dimension will be there simply because there is conflict of a moral nature from the very beginning and, furthermore, the secret of its origins can be found in the Freudian captation of *das Ding*, as he dealt with it in the 'Project'.

Where will we find an ethics of Psychoanalysis if the very fabric of existence is based on a paradox—dying to enjoy life yet living ourselves to death? As Lacan says:

> The ethical limits of Psychoanalysis will coincide with the limits of its practice, its practice is only a preliminary to moral action as such—the so-called action being the one through which we enter the Real. (Lacan 1992: 22)

In other words psychoanalysis will lead one to the door of moral choice—but how do we explain the fact that a subject's impulses may draw him elsewhere? Freud's answer to this problem will be different from that of Aristotle.

We are seeking a truth in psychoanalysis but it is a particular truth. It is a truth that will be found in a hiding place in the subject and the form of its articulation is a *Wunsch* or 'wish'. This wish has its genesis in the experience of pleasure or pain. Lacan analyses it in the following manner:

> We find it in the form that we have categorised as a regressive infantile unrealistic phase characterised by a thought abandoned to desire—by the desire taken to be a reality. (Lacan 1992: 24)

It is, in fact, the truth of the thought of desire. We are in the field of *das Ding*.

If *das Ding* is the motor behind the real—Lacan puts it at the very core—at the centre of the Real—it is in fact the Real par excellence—then the question becomes how can the human subject be ethical or, to put it in Lacanian terms, 'given our condition as men what can we do to act in the right way' (Lacan 1992: 19). How can we draw upon The Thing to help us act in the *good* way? Is the very question itself a rhetorical one? Each person must discover it—deal with it, circumvent it in his own way—do the best he can—this is partly the reason why, I question, whether there can be an Ethics of Psychoanalysis.

What is this *das Ding* that has such profound implications for the human subject? Freud makes reference on four principal occasions to *das Ding* in the 'Project'.[1] He shows in this work how the psychical apparatus functions in such a way as to restore the state of inertia—of constancy. It is principally a hedonistic apparatus obeying the pleasure principle. It is with the introduction of *Begierde*—of 'desire'—or, to be more precise, of 'yearning', linked to the *Not des Lebens*—to the 'necessities or dangers of life'—when the infant is in a state of distress—that certain questions arise. Freud states that a 'specific action' (Freud 1950: 318) is needed to remove this distress and that the infant is incapable of bringing about this specific action by himself.

I will partly paraphrase Freud here. At first, the human organism is incapable of bringing about this specific action. It takes place by extraneous help when the attention of the experienced person is drawn by the child's screaming. This scream for Freud acquires a function of the highest importance—that of communication and this initial helplessness of human beings is the primal source of all moral motives.

We are already in the field of *das Ding*. Here with the notion of *Begierde*—of 'yearning'—there is anticipation which from then on is linked to the idea of the function of the other. When the other—the helpful person—has carried out the specific action the infant is of course relieved of his pain, and Freud tells us that this 'total event constitutes an experience of satisfaction' (Freud 1950: 318). Freud informs us in neurophysiological terms of the three consequences which ensue from this. What follows is a psychoanalytical reading of these terms:

1) The agency of distress in the infant is brought to an end. This occurs not by the real perception of an object—but by the anticipation of finding that object again—to verify if it is still there in reality. This anticipation then is a hallucinatory one. Lacan says about this 'the world of perception is represented by Freud as dependent on that fundamental hallucination without which there would be no attention available' (Lacan 1992: 53). This bringing to an end of the distress happens after the fact—after the scream—therefore at the level of the secondary process. All the distress had in fact occurred before the scream so that the scream is what gives it support in the Symbolic Order—to paraphrase Lacan.

2) The second effect of this 'experience of satisfaction' is that the perception of the Object (based on this fundamental hallucination) arouses vigorous interest in the infant to try and find that object again—this experience of satisfaction is not in fact an object—it is a thing but it's not any old thing, it is *the Thing*. As a corollary to this 'the specific action' which was the action of the helper becomes the specific action of the infant in his attempts to find *das Ding*. It does not seem to be based on any kind of primordial identification but is simply, as Freud says, 'a reflex action' (Freud 1950: 317-9). The infant's specific action then becomes a way of reproducing the object over and over again. This implies that he will always be missing something—we are perhaps in the world of the Real because we are in the world of the truly missed encounter—but we are also in the world of faith—because what is that yearning to verify the object if not an act of faith?

3) The third consequence of this (experience of satisfaction) is that the state of inertia is restored so that the subject finds that ideas fit together in his thoughts. These are unconscious thoughts, of course—how these thought-processes reach consciousness moving from representation to representation would be the subject matter of another paper.

The characteristic of the *Begierde,* Freud tells us, is to verify the image of the memory even to the point of hallucinating it (Freud 1950: 319, 381). Freud brings in here the function of the ego—it serves as a regulatory apparatus as well as a function to ensure inhibition and defence in so far as it distinguishes if the signs of perception are those of an image of a memory or those of an object—in other words, if they are signs of reality. We note from this that the ego is an unconscious one following the pleasure principle, and yet it's that very same pleasure principle which regulates reality.

I would now like to go through the four instances of *das Ding* in the 'Project'.

Freud mentions *das Ding* firstly in relation to the Ego (Freud 1950: 328)—ensuring the reality of the object wished for. The Ego is seen as having a function of inhibition but also because of its relationship with *das Ding* it has a participatory function with all the consequences of *das Ding*. It would be going too far to say that *das Ding* is incorporated into the Ego but, as Freud says: 'There is a resemblance between the nucleus of the Ego and The Thing' (Freud 1950: 328).

If, as sometimes happens, the wish and the perception of it concurs then that is fine—'the discharge is successful' (Freud 1950: 328). But—if the wish is there and there is only a perception which does not tally with it wholly but only in part, what happens then? Freud tells us that the world of yearning—is *total* yearning—all of the subject's energy goes into making this perception happen—but he also informs us that there is always a discrepancy between wishes and perception; they never tally uniformly—in other words there is never correspondence between the wish and the perception. Wishes are all-encompassing and so is the world of perception. As the poet William Blake says: 'If the doors of perception were cleared everything would appear to man as it is—infinite' (Bloom & Trilling 1973: 40).

There is an inherent break, rupture—disagreement at the heart of the organism. Freud then searches for a way of completing the similarity into an identity—of making wishes and perception coincide. In other words, he searches for a way of trying to understand the Real. What he does, in his own words, is to dissect the perceptual complex into a component portion Neurone A which remains the same and a second component Neurone B—which for the most part varies. Language—he tells us—will call Neurone A 'The Thing', and Neurone B 'its activity or attribute'—in short, its predicate (cf. Freud 1950: 328).

The first thing that can be said about this is that there is something there which is unchanging, constant, immobile. The Real is that which will always escape total comprehension—total judgement—and yet *das Ding* will later inform language about this judgement because, as Freud says, language will call Neurone A 'The Thing', so that Neurone A is what it is and Neurone B is out of the fact of Neurone A, but not like it. We can then say that the Symbolic is a predicate of the Real and that the Symbolic process itself is woven into it. This will have implications for any possible ethics of psychoanalysis, because where the Real meets the Symbolic there is the possibility for a little bit of reality by which we can try to get our bearings. In fact, in his 1925 article 'Negation', Freud has shown that the very condition of reality-testing itself is that it is based on the loss of an object which once brought real satisfaction (Freud 1925c: 283). Kant used his judgement here in this space—of The Thing—to call forth his imperative to do one's duty. Everyone will march to his own tune here, depending on the remnants left over from the after-effects of the scream. In other words each person, it seems to me, will be obliged to answer for himself what is in him that makes this loss possible so that his desire can emerge from it. There can be no standard answer even for a psychoanalyst.

The second mention of *das Ding* in the 'Project' (Freud 1950: 331) is very important to outline in detail because it shows the essentially conflictual position of the human subject with regard to his own satisfaction, and I think we can locate here the archaic origins of *jouissance.* Here Freud emphasises the consequence of situating *das Ding* in the complex of perception and, he says:

> ...let us suppose that the object which furnishes the perception resembles the subject—a fellow human being. If so the theoretical interest taken in it is also explained by the fact that an object like this was simultaneously the subject's first satisfying object and further his first hostile one as well as his sole helping power. For this reason it is in relation to another that a human being learns to cognise. (Freud 1950: 331)

Before all this can happen two conditions must be fulfilled. These are:-

- a perception arises which does not coincide with the wish;

- what happens then is that the infant wishes with all his heart to recognise this image, so that it may be possible to find a way through it to the longed-for image.

Freud is here showing how desire can create something out of nothing. All our roads lead us back the same way it seems—to that first wish for an object which was never there. In fact, Freud shows that it's only when things don't work that the activity of thought is set in motion. So the wish which doesn't succeed gives rise to a thought which in turn gives rise to a desire which in turn is taken for reality—

that is what Freud seems to be saying. This object is searched for by the subject to fulfil desire—as Lacan says: 'It's a probing form of progress that seeks points of reference in relation to the world of desires' (Lacan 1992: 52).

Written in to the very notion of satisfaction there is pain because, as Freud himself states, the wished-for object was never there in the first place. This loss and subsequent re-finding of the object is of the very nature of *jouissance*—in every satisfaction there is pain and repetition of satisfaction in every pain—this is the way things are. These endless horizons of *jouissance* played out by an object which is no object—this *Ding*—Freud tells us—will make an impression by its constant structure—is in fact my *nebenmensch*—my 'neighbour'. In other words, it is from the other that we learn to recognise ourselves—in the beginning the other is I and yet not I and vice versa. It is from memories of one's own body that one learns to recognise otherness. *Das Ding* is the constancy behind this. How terribly close we all are and yet how hostile? The only difference between me and my neighbour is a space, until the signifier will imprint its signifying difference. Freud continues:

> ...other perceptions of the object too—if for instance he screams will awaken the memory of the subject's own screaming and at the same time of his own experience of pain. (Freud 1950: 331)

'Love your neighbour as yourself', the Gospel exhorts us—but if your neighbour is really only your neighbour in this unbearable architecture of *jouissance*, what then? Outside this centre of myself which I loathe is there someone nearer to me whom I am asked to love? The Thing is the subject's other, that much is certain.

Desire, then, seems to be always in relation to a lure, so that this neighbour could indeed be part of my own reflection—as Lacan has pointed out—and moreover the striking thing for the Freudian formation is that he is *hostile*. Where would we begin to formulate an ethics around that?

Freud has shown how primeval this hostility is, and so it seems to me that *das Ding* brings to light the whole question of evil. If it does this then it also raises the question of sublimation. '*Das Ding* is the place of desire whether it be perverse or sublimated', Lacan says (Lacan 1992: 110). Sublimation consists in taking the lack—the gap—and creating something new with it. Is not the example of the infant wishing with all his heart to get to his desire—is not this a Freudian exercise in sublimation? The infant here is going round The Thing so that he can join with Lacan in saying that sublimation 'raises an object to the dignity of The Thing' (Lacan 1992: 112). This is exactly what the infant does. This child knows that he can never know the Thing as Thing and so the drive is provided with a satisfaction different to its aim, which is Freud's own definition of sublimation. But as we are in the field of desire no one can know for sure which way the dice will turn.

The third mention of *das Ding* is also an important one (Freud 1950: 366) because here for the first time speech is used to communicate the infant's distress to another and so we see how the speech action is made part of the specific action. The very sound of the scream together with the image of the object emphasises that object as a hostile one. Freud says: 'The information of one's own scream serves to characterise that object' (Freud 1950: 366). The scream comes to inform and this information will help to make memories conscious. Our first conscious memories are always of an unpleasurable nature according to Freud. So—The Thing becomes the master of memory. There is no escaping it. This Thing will remain part of the storehouse of knowledge that is a human being and 'after such knowledge what forgiveness' as the poet T. S. Eliot asks (Eliot 1963: 122). I wonder if it is here that the function of the father will enter? To help stop the flow of this impossible *jouissance,* or at least to turn it around—otherwise the scream will hold us in its thrall. Surely the working of sublimation is to turn Death around? The father's function is closely linked to this in that it helps open the door to a wider reality than that of being enveloped by the Thing. Perhaps an ethics of psychoanalysis should begin with an understanding of the position and function of the father?

Where is the hope in all this? It seems to me that hope comes along with the last mention by Freud of *das Ding* (Freud 1950: 383). 'But let it not be hope for the wrong thing'—again to quote T.S. Eliot (Eliot 1963)—and this will be my conclusion.

When Freud talks about practical thought he is in fact talking about desire, because it (practical thought) does not seek an end in itself but seeks to 'discover along what paths it will lead to the putting into play of the original wish' (Freud 1950: 376).

He postulates that when this activity of thought (in other words, this desire) has been set in motion then the wished-for state can be attained without regard to the reality of the situation at any given moment. In other words, the human subject can climb mountains of great magnitude. But—Freud is quite clear on this—this can only happen when The Thing has been firmly put in its place—if we include it in our calculations—take responsibility for it—make friends with it—only then can desire find its pathway. Desire can save us, because it contains within itself the possibility of forgiveness. Because of The Thing the human subject is liable to make a mistake—to err. The existence of The Thing can lead to 'mistakes in judgement or faults in the premises' (Freud 1950: 384).

Once we understand, we can forgive—and forgiveness could be one possible exit.

Freud's *das Ding* is the trajectory of a psychoanalysis, but the story does not end there. The question then becomes not whether one has succeeded in being more moral or indeed ethical, and not whether those concepts are now redundant—far from it—the question then becomes, has the experience been profound enough to understand the echoes and the implications of a final analysis?

Notes

1 See Freud 1950: 328, 331, 366, 383.

ON THE ORIGINS OF PSYCHIC STRUCTURE: A CASE-STUDY REVISITED ON THE BASIS OF FREUD'S 'PROJECT'

Gertrudis Van De Vijver

Introduction

One of the most striking points in Freud's approach to psychic phenomena, is that he conceives of them—basically—in materialist, dynamic and structural terms. Psychic phenomena are taken to be of a material nature, and are apprehended on the basis of specific, concrete mechanisms. The dynamic aspect refers to the fact that matter can only be shaped by a particular history. The structuralist aspect refers to the more or less fixed results of this particular history: the particular pathways which were formed, which continue to be formed throughout a lifetime, and which determine subsequent behaviour.

Various authors in this volume have stressed that the basic elements of this materialist, structuralist and dynamic approach were already present in Freud's pre-analytical writings.[1] Some go so far as to state that, in his later works, and in his metapsychological texts in particular, this dynamic, evolutionary approach shifts towards a purely structuralist approach, and comes close to what is described as 'psychological reductionism'. This means that psychic phenomena and functioning are reduced or restricted purely to *representational* functionings.

It is certainly tempting to describe the history of psychoanalysis in terms of its oscillations between evolutionary and dynamic accounts of the psyche, on the one hand, and structuralist accounts, on the other. For instance, in his return to Freud, Lacan focuses primarily on the structuralist aspects which were quite clearly present in all of Freud's texts (see also Trobas 1999).

I shall not, however, enter into the theoretical discussion of reductionism, as related to structuralism and evolutionism. The question I wish to address here is twofold. Firstly, I will try to show that a structuralist account of psychic phenomena has major advantages over a purely formal account of psychic—and, more specifically, *cognitive* phenomena. Secondly, I will tackle the question of the *material* genesis of structure. More concretely, I wish to trace the implications of a dynamic and materialist viewpoint on the origins of psychic structure for a theory of higher order psychic phenomena—that is, a theory of cognitive and linguistic phenomena.

In so doing I will arrive at the question of the relation between structure and embodiment. Today questions related to this issue also crop up in other fields, such as cognitive science and artificial life (Hendriks-Jansen 1996), phenomenology (Sheets-Johnstone 1996) and biology (Salthe 1993). In most of these fields, which are experiencing the shortcomings of a formal, a-historical view of the psyche and cognition, the need for a dynamic and embodied approach to structure and cognition makes itself clearly felt. However, the lack of specific mechanisms, and the absence of particular case-studies which might form the basis of such a theory, is also manifest.

I believe that the early writings of Freud—in particular the 'Project' (1950)—contain useful insights and pertinent questions on this subject. Freud's distinction between understanding and judging, which he introduces in the 'Project', is particularly useful for highlighting some methodological difficulties related to the concepts of structure and embodiment. The way in which Freud deals with this issue in the 'Project' enables us to realise that the mechanism of *identification* complicates the notion of embodiment and leads to a fundamentally interactionist or constructivist viewpoint on psychic structure—that is, a viewpoint in which the *fellow human being* plays a central role. Every self-recognition or self-description, every acquisition of a body, is mediated by the other.

I shall demonstrate this by examining the interesting case-study of a young boy, named Herbert (Sterba 1933). The case-study dates from the thirties, but is quite relevant to the present volume, because it deals with a boy who was diagnosed as psychotic by his analyst, Edita Sterba, at a time when the theory of psychosis had not yet been developed within a Freudian framework. Ironically, then, not only am I using a case-study of a young psychotic boy dating from a 'pre-psychotic' period, but also a pre-analytical text—the 'Project'—in order to qualify some of my explanations. Above all, I aim to pose the question of structure and embodiment, in relation to the current state of affairs in cognitive science, artificial life, and the biological theory of evolution. In addition, I believe that psychoanalytic theory itself, having worked through its Lacanian structuralist heritage, could benefit from adopting some of the more materialist and dynamic aspects of the early Freudian works. A dynamic structuralist theory of the psyche is certainly one of the most interesting directions to pursue in a variety of disciplines.

On the necessity of a structuralist viewpoint

When a young child asks: 'Do nightingales make night?', one might easily presume that this is a typical expression of a particular stage of language development. And when a child of about the same age asks: 'What are five minutes, compared to eternity?', one can only be filled with admiration at such a capacity for abstract ideas. However, if the same child says, when language is already well-mastered: 'I can't eat "whipped cream", because otherwise, I will be whipped'; or, 'I need a first class ticket, because I am a first class boy'; or else 'I don't want to put on the green coat, I *am* a big boy, and I don't want to be a frog, I don't want to put on the green coat', then one can quite legitimately begin to wonder *why* he is talking in such a bizarre manner.

All these examples, except for the first, come from a five-year old boy, Herbert, who mastered the Austrian language perfectly at fourteen months, and who, from this early age onwards, enjoyed reading encyclopaedias and books, learning and memorising their contents at an amazing speed. Other children asked themselves: 'Is this a child?', and wondered: 'How can he be so smart yet at the same time be so stupid?'.

This case-study, written more than sixty years ago by the Viennese child analyst, Edita Sterba, is entitled '*Ein abnormes Kind: aus seiner Krankengeschichte und Behandlung*' (Sterba 1933).[2] Sterba diagnosed the boy as suffering from infantile psychosis.

Herbert's story fills one with admiration and astonishment. For, indeed, who would not want to be able to read and memorise so quickly, or to be a mathematical wonder? Yet, at the same time, who would want to be afraid of eating whipped cream, wearing green coats, seeing keyholes or saying dirty words for fear of becoming them? This was the fate of the young boy, for whom a social life was practically impossible.

The problem with psychosis, however, is that one does not become psychotic by force of will. The intentional formulation, 'who would not want to...', is therefore out of place. How, then, ought we to understand why and how such strange behaviour can occur? This is one of the mysteries of mental illness, but it is also a mystery of psychic phenomena in general. The question to be asked is: how do people develop into different modalities of being, or into different structures? In other words, what are the material conditions that account for the fact that some children are structured to behave and talk strangely, while others are apparently quite comfortable with language and daily life?

If I use a case like Herbert's as a point of departure, it is because it possesses various remarkable aspects which, in my opinion, can serve to disentangle some issues with regard to the origin of higher order psychical phenomena.

Firstly, if one wishes to deal with the origin of linguistic and cognitive phenomena, one must also deal with the origin of structure. The reasons for this will become clear in the course of this paper, but one question might begin to enlighten us: can we consider the origin of Herbert's formal encyclopaedic knowledge *separately* from his rather inflexible and correct language manipulation, and from his bizarre way of embodying this knowledge?

Secondly, using a psychotic structure as a point of departure has a major advantage: it prevents an all too hasty interpretation of what goes on or appears in the clinical picture. Herbert's behaviour and language are far from familiar; they drive his mother to despair, his younger brother into a cruel rivalry, and then confront his therapist with major puzzles of human knowledge. Psychosis is a perfect safeguard against a common-sense understanding, a safeguard which, I think, is badly needed today by science, particularly the cognitive sciences. Common-sense frequently leads to a semblance of understanding, when we are confronted with the familiar. But when this semblance of understanding is backed up by a vague and distant ideal—an ideal of the perfect language, of perfect normality, of the most appropriate cognition—it frequently leads to a complete denial, even a scotomisation, of that which is unfamiliar. Philosophers of understanding are frequently experts in this, although I would far prefer them to be experts in *astonishment*.

I shall reap some elements from Herbert's case, and will sow them again—so to speak—as 'seeds of astonishment' in the field of psychoanalysis and cognitive research. I will then relate these to some impasses in classical cognitive science, but also hope to point at some possible solutions.

On systems which are closed with regard to meaning

At first sight, one might be tempted to compare Herbert to a computer. One might consider him as a perfect example of a system which is closed with regard to its semantics (Petitot 1990: 140). If we consider Herbert's ability to memorise information, and to use and reproduce it correctly afterwards, as well his formal capacities, his grammatically correct way of speaking, and his ability to count very quickly, then it becomes quite evident that he is closer to a high-performance computer than most humans, who handle information in a rather more flexible but not fully reliable manner. If we consider, moreover, that it is difficult for Herbert to establish a connection with the outer world, or to establish a relation of 'aboutness' or 'directedness' to his environment, we might come to the conclusion that, in his case, the ability to process information and to manipulate symbols does not necessarily imply that he has access to the semantic properties of mental representations.

Among these 'semantic properties', Fodor lists those of: 'being true, of having referents... the property of being representations *of the environment*.' (Fodor 1982: 283). Herbert may compute information in a highly reliable way, but this does not entail he has no access to the semantic properties to which Fodor refers. This would over-simplify the matter, the reason being that the assumption of a dichotomy between Herbert's formal capacities and his way of being in the world is inappropriate.

Indeed, when one observes the clinical picture, the impossibility and the irrelevance of isolating Herbert's formal qualities become very clear. Sterba suggests that Herbert has so much energy at his disposal to deal with purely intellectual or formal matters, precisely because he is physically so ill-adapted to the outer world. Normally, people waste time and lose track of things, because their attention shifts and spreads over many things at once. Herbert, however, displays no such problem with attention. In a sense, he is aware neither of his body nor of the behaviour of people in his surroundings. For a number of reasons, unrelated to physical disability, Herbert is unable to dress, to wash or to eat decently like other boys of his age; he cannot venture down the street alone without endangering his life.

I will not dwell on the fact that Sterba draws on the energetic terminology which was fashionable at that time. What she rightly stresses, however, is the inherent link between Herbert's substantial formal capacities and his lack of bodily understanding. If he is able to pursue formal cognition with endless enthusiasm and concentration, this is because of his particular embodiment of this type of knowledge.

Formal approaches to cognition

The idea that Herbert has 'energy at his disposal' for formal matters because he wastes no time with his body, is clearly not an issue in the philosophical tradition, nor, I gather, in mainstream cognitive sciences. It is a question that simply cannot be dealt with in this context. It is easy to show how far removed philosophy and cognitive sciences are from such questions, and how difficult it is to address them once one has taken some basically divergent theoretical decisions.

Take, for instance, one of the founders of the formal study of language and cognition—Gotlob Frege.[3] What is remarkable about Frege, is that he clearly had the ambition to formalise natural language, as far and as faithfully as possible. To him formalising language meant revealing its logical structure, with the clear aim of ascertaining that from true premises—always, by necessity—follow true conclusions. For Frege, natural language can, to a certain extent, be compared to the eye: within certain limits it serves us very well. However, the perfect formal language envisaged by Frege would function as a microscope; it would not allow us to have a global overview all of the time, but would allow us to determine with high precision exactly what follows from what (Kenny 1995: 13).

Although Frege's proposition has generally met with acceptance throughout this century—consider, for instance, the examples of analytical philosophy, or of classical cognitive science—it is nevertheless important to outline as clearly as possible its presuppositions and its implications. Frege firmly believed that a systematic or formal study of language was a prerequisite for the development of true knowledge, and that the formal language should not be formalisation for formalisation's sake. For Frege, the formalisation of natural language is *formalisation with a view to truth*. In other words, the form is what permits the transmission—in a very precise way—of content. The form is what permits us to deal systematically with a content. To quote Montaigne: '*La forme, c'est la chair même de la pensée*'.

However, in his articles on content (for instance 'Function and Object' or 'On Sense and Reference'), Frege simply presupposes that those 'who are sufficiently familiar with the language' will understand the content—that is, the *sense*—of words and sentences. As a logician who wishes to develop a formal theory of scientific knowledge, he also presupposes a reference.[4] From this we can deduce three points: firstly, Frege attributes no importance to the question of the origin of meaning; secondly, he does not believe that understanding could be quite intimately linked to psychical structures; thirdly, the body plays an insignificant role in the development of a meaningful relation to the world.

Of course, one can hardly expect Frege to believe that a theory of language *should* deal with these things. Indeed, the Fregean project developed in full resistance to psychologism, and to what might be called the 'subjective' side of meaning. The least one can say is that any kind of naturalistic endeavour was at odds with the aims Frege set himself.

Even so, the problem persisted. To the extent that Frege believed his formalisation of language was to be developed with a view to truth, he 'objectified' meaning and simply took it for granted that people who were sufficiently familiar with the language would be able to understand or grasp the meanings of words and sentences. This led to the very ambiguous status of his theory of knowledge, and of what he meant by 'a referent' or 'an object'. In other words, it led to the completely unproblematised 'empirical' dimensions of language and cognition.

The classical viewpoint in cognitive sciences reflects a similar approach. Cognitive processes are seen as computational processes. They can be described as 'formal' in that they apply to representations solely by virtue of the form of the representations. Cognitive processes can also be described as 'symbolic', however, in that they are defined by means of representations—that is, by means of things that represent something, that refer to something (cf. Fodor 1982). It is evident, however, that a theory of cognition, even if its first objective is to make things work, cannot be considered as a true theory of cognition if it is a purely formal matter. This leads us into discussions about the status of representations, the parallelism between the syntactical structure of a representation and its physical counterpart (Newell 1980; Engel 1992: 11, 30-34), and the status of psychological explanations—which are causal explanations based on inferential processes.

To summarise the most striking features of this formal-symbolic approach: (i) it does not consider as important the fact that cognitive systems are internally structured objects; (ii) it does not account for the fact that the internal structure somehow determines the way of being in the world; (iii) it does not take into account the fact that internal structures are formed by a particular history, in which interfere not only biological mechanisms—such as those related to perception—but also mechanisms related to the use of language by fellow human beings; and, finally, (iv) it does not deal with the embodiment of cognition, interpreted from a structuralist and historical point of view.

Herbert's challenge

I do not mean to suggest that a formalist-symbolic approach is irrelevant when compared with a structuralist one. My concern here is with purposes and priorities: how far can either of these two approaches lead us, and of what kind of linguistic and cognitive phenomena can they provide an account?

For instance, Herbert is evidently much more than a computer which reliably fulfils certain formal tasks. He not only uses language in a grammatically correct manner, but in a way that is contextually rather flexible and apt. For instance, when his teacher urges him to put on his shoes more rapidly (that is, in less than five minutes) Herbert has no difficulty replying: 'What are five minutes, compared to eternity?'. Additionally, he experiences no problems in talking, adequately, in many different contexts, and after only a couple of months of therapy, he was able to abandon the use of the third-person and began to speak of himself in the first-person.[5]

One must admit that Herbert is able to conceive of words as having a *function*; in other words, he is evidently aware that words inherently refer to something else. He is evidently able to acknowledge the indicative function, or the sign-function of words. A sign, in the Peircean sense, is 'something which stands to somebody for something in some respect or capacity' (cited in Buchler 1955: 125); a sign is 'a difference that makes a difference' (Bateson 1972).

Why, then, on certain occasions, does Herbert *not* evince this capacity, but declines to use words in their capacity as sign-function? I am referring to the previously mentioned example of the 'whipped cream'. This particular clinical phenomenon has incited many clinicians to conjecture that psychotic subjects attribute the status of 'things' to words or language fragments.

Words are things

Sterba states that sentences such as: 'I can't eat whipped cream, otherwise I may be whipped', or: 'If we can say "*Her-vorragend*", why can't we say "*Frau-vorragend*"?', show that, on such occasions, Herbert lost the *content* of the words 'whipped cream' or '*her-vorragend*'. She suggests that Herbert must have been in the possession of the content at a certain moment, but somehow lost track of it. The 'somehow' is not always unclear to Sterba, considering Herbert's particular history, in which some painful, traumatic events related to intrusions into his body took place. However, I shall not deal with the role of trauma in the development of psychosis.

Instead, I would like to focus on the idea of having a relation to a content at a certain moment, and losing it at another. To me, this is quite problematic and seems a rather inadequate way of interpreting what is going on. Even if the clinical picture in psychosis is well known, it is easy to say or to observe that words are things for someone, but much less easy to actually understand what this entails.

What this idea basically suggests is that words are treated literally or, as is sometimes stated, 'materially'. In this case, words are taken to be indivisible and, as such, they are treated as entities. Hence, there is nothing behind words; a word is merely 'thing-hood'. If Herbert refuses to eat whipped cream, he refuses to eat the word 'whipped'. If he fears eating whipped cream, he fears experiencing the consequences that he associates with the thing-word 'whipped'. Similarly, if he fears verbalising the parts of his body, he therefore fears that something might happen to those parts, that he might loose or hurt them.

However by saying that 'there is nothing behind a word' for Herbert, I do not wish to suggest that it has *no* meaning, *no* content. Herbert is not a machine that refuses to eat physically instantiated symbols. In this case, the question becomes *which* kinds of meaning does he not grasp; in *which* contexts does he fail to manipulate symbols correctly?

Freud's 'Project': understanding and judging

One of Freud's ideas, which he introduced more than a hundred years ago, holds—for me—an enduring fascination. Even though it might require refinement and specification today, I believe that it still has a significant impact upon discussions relating to the origins of the psychical structure and the notion of embodiment.

In his 'A Project for a Scientific Psychology' (1950a), Freud attempts to describe psychological states and processes on the basis of the *quantitative* workings of material particles. In the chapter on remembering and judging, which deals with the particular case of perceiving and knowing a fellow human being, he writes:

> Thus the complex of the fellow human being falls apart into two components, of which one makes an impression by its constant structure and stays together as a *thing*, while the other can be *understood* by the activity of memory—that is, can be traced back to information from [the subject's] own body. This dissection of a perceptual complex is described as *cognising* it; it involves a *judgement* and when this last aim has been attained it comes to an end. (Freud 1950a: 331)

Understanding

The first intriguing aspect of this excerpt is the idea that what one can understand is that which can be traced back to memories of movements of the subject's own body. Freud explained this in slightly more detail a few lines earlier:

> Let us suppose that the object which furnishes the perception resembles the subject—a *fellow human-being*... Then the perceptual complexes proceeding from this fellow human-being will in part be new and non-comparable—his *features*, for instance, in the visual sphere; but other visual perceptions—e.g. those of the movements of his hand—will coincide in the subject with memories of quite similar visual impressions of his own, of his own body, [memories] which are associated with memories of movements experienced by himself. Other perceptions of the object too—if, for instance, he screams—will awaken the memory of this [the subject's] own screaming and at the same time of his own experiences of pain. (Freud 1950a: 331)

It is quite remarkable that, according to Freud, understanding something implies that one must have lived it physically. Similar bodily experiences, or memories of those experiences, are thus *a prerequi-*

site for understanding. In other words, one is only able to understand that which finds resonance in the body. This is the only way I can grasp the meaning of Freud's term 'understanding' in this context. I am quite sympathetic to this idea that understanding does not go further than that—namely, that it is a private, material, non-cognitive matter.

Does this imply that the words whose content Herbert 'lost' (as Sterba puts it—for instance, the 'whipped cream') are therefore totally excluded from Herbert's bodily experience? I think this is clearly not the case. Herbert may well have lost the content in language, but certainly not in his body: this is illustrated vividly by the way that Herbert has a good bodily reason for not wanting to eat whipped cream. In other words, he has a very lucid understanding of the word! To him, the word is pregnant with bodily experiences, related to visits to the ear-clinic and various kinds of painful intrusions into his body.

The fact that 'words are things', then, does not imply that Herbert's bodily experiences lack meaning or memory. Herbert's body grasps the dangers of being whipped only too well. What it does imply, on the other hand, is that Herbert is not able to subscribe to the fact that a word is a word, and that, as such, it can stand for *many* things; indeed, a word can refer to *anything*. It is precisely this fundamental indeterminacy that Herbert is unable to recognise. It is a mystery how a system can genuinely *recognise* the sign-function. Applying and manipulating words in their indicative function, is quite different from actually recognising this function.

It is noticeable that all the difficulties Herbert experiences are, in one way or another connected with his body. They are all related to his material way of being in the world. What clearly transpires from this case, then, is that Herbert is incapable of saying anything about the particular inscriptions in the body. To use Freud's terminology, one could conjecture that Herbert is not able to make a judgement. The moment his being is concerned, he is unable to grasp the predicate and the thing in a judgement. In this sense, it is impossible for him to know something, to arrive at knowledge related to his body or to himself. If there is disturbance, it is disturbance in relation to the way in which he can grasp himself in a judgement, or, more precisely, there is disturbance in his ability to identify himself with something or somebody.

This brings us to the second theme formulated by Freud, concerning that which possesses a constant structure and stays together as 'a thing'. The question here is whether we can *understand* a thing, for if that which impresses by its structure remains forever outside our understanding—as Freud suggests—then what kind of relation can be developed with it? This brings us to one of the most important questions for various disciplines today, from cybernetics to artificial life and biology: the question of what knowledge we can develop concerning systems which 'stay together as a thing'?

Beyond understanding: identification and embodiment

In the passage quoted above Freud states that to arrive at knowledge, one must make a connection between the thing and the predicate, between that which can be understood and that which lies beyond understanding. Freud's question was concerned with how one can know fellow human beings and oneself. Or, more generally speaking, is it possible to know systems that stay together as a thing, *as* things that stay together? Human beings, as organisms, have an internal structure, which implies that they 'make an impression by their constant structure and that they stay together as a thing'. Hence, one can never have an experience, or a memory of an experience, of such a being in its totality. It is impossible to understand fellow human beings *as* structured beings. Instead, *identification* is the response to questions such as 'What am I?' and 'Who am I?'. It is identification which enables one to make a distinction between inside and outside (cf. Van de Vijver 1996b).

Freud's answer to these questions is that a little child cannot understand the fellow human being, and therefore can only identify with him. I think we could apply this reasoning to everything 'that stays together as a thing'—that is, to *all* autonomous, living, self-organising beings. Indeed, as I hope to demonstrate, Herbert himself suggests something similar.

However, let us first examine identification, which is the way in which an organism succeeds in recognising itself, in building a representation of itself, or in giving itself a place in the functioning of the outer world, on the basis of an interaction with his surroundings. As perceiving systems, living beings do not stand in a relation of cognitive self-awareness, because the organism has to recognise itself in the stimulus. As Dalto states: 'The factor capable of showing it to itself is for Freud the constant stimulus, which implies that the organism can only recognise its unity by identifying with the latter. This implies the fact that when I say "I", this does not only refer to my organic individuality, but conversely to that same organic individuality in so far as it is strictly equivalent to the perceptual mirror in which it sees itself' (Dalto 1999). This is what René Thom and many other ethologists suggest when they state that the moment the predator chases the prey, the predator *is* the prey.

For human beings, identification also contains this mirror-like aspect, leading to what is called the identification with the image. I find it quite mysterious that a human being, upon seeing itself in the mirror, should come to the conclusion that what it sees there, outside itself, *is* itself. One always identifies with what one is not. Indeed, Freud himself is very succinct on this point when he writes, in the opening pages of 'Instincts and Their Vicissitudes': 'all that I can directly withdraw from, this is not me; on the contrary, all that I cannot directly withdraw from, this is me' (Freud 1915a: 119). What I cannot escape, then, is me. In other words, if it is a thing that stays together and that impresses by its constant structure, it can be me.

It should be observed that in some cases, such as that of Herbert, this mechanism does not function. Although Herbert's behaviour in front of the mirror was not described in the case, it is well known that most psychotic subjects have immense difficulties with mirrors, because they are not able to recognise themselves and consequently experience the image as a major threat to their own being.

However, the peculiarity of humans is that they are not just organisms. They do not restrict themselves to imaginary identification. Humans are born in language, and most of the time assume the idea that words can represent them, thereby immediately experiencing the inadequacy of words which—in fact—can never fully represent them. In this sense, it could be said that entering language implies that one accepts the fundamental impossibility of making the word and the thing coincide. Hence, the way of being in language expresses something of one's way of being in the world, in a bodily, spatial and temporal manner. The 'biological' is a re-appropriation in *language* by beings that are produced in and through language. I could thus paraphrase Maxine Sheets-Johnstone's statement: 'Animals are topological beings: they move as they shape and they shape as they move' (Sheets-Johnstone 1996) as follows: 'Humans are topological beings: they *speak* as they shape and they shape as they *speak*'.

The particular material conditions which are necessary for being in language remain, however, unknown, although it seems certain that the 'fellow human-being' and his way of being in language have a determinative effect. I think it would be interesting to consider the fellow human-being in terms of the perturbations he effects upon the biological structure of the organism. The other perturbs—in a more or less drastic way—the biological rhythms of the organism; he perturbs the various productions of the child by interpreting them; he perturbs by being absent or present. Thus we have two interacting structures: one that is in language (in a particular way), and another that is not yet language and which is under-interpreted and over-interpreted at the same time. For instance, the mother inevitably adds her own meaning by interpreting the behaviour of the child (over-interpretation), yet—just as inevitably—fails to interpret adequately the child's behaviour (under-interpretation). Freud arrives at a similar analysis in the 'Project'. However, it seems to me that we are far from having stipulated the conditions or the precise mechanisms which are at work here.

As far as the question of embodiment is concerned, Herbert's case offers two distinct advantages: it obliges us to conceive of embodiment in very concrete terms, and it illustrates that the assumption or acknowledgement of the fact that one has a body, is very different from the simple biological fact of displaying organismic unity or structure.

Herbert demonstrates clearly that his body is not something unified, something with a border, which therefore stays together. It is not something about which he can say 'this is my body, and these are the various parts of it'. His body is something that can be transpierced at any moment; it can fall apart, and be penetrated from all sides. Herbert constantly fears being invaded, for instance, by water (he does not dare take a bath without having shoes on); by particular types of food, which can make holes in his mouth; and by doctors, who can come at any moment and destroy him. The quite natural way in which other children talk about themselves, their bodily experiences and their pains and pleasures, are completely alien to Herbert.

All of this is reflected in Herbert's language. For instance, he refuses to name the parts of his body, for doing so would mean taking the risk of being destroyed. He has memories of various painful intrusions, but cannot express them. Hence, Herbert can only build protective shells around his lack of being.[6] The clinical picture shows that Herbert is deeply involved in every word concerning his body. It shows that words are *things* to him; and to verbalise them would involve too much danger.

Likewise, Herbert also refuses to acknowledge the fact that he is a boy. He says that there is nothing between his legs, that he is a girl. This is what is most comfortable for him, because it means that he has nothing to loose. His erections cause him extreme anxiety and lead him to deny all that is related to them, to refuse to talk about them, and to construct a very sophisticated discourse with many new words which aims at totally avoiding what actually causes him these troubles.

It is obvious that Herbert fails to grasp himself through an image of his body, or through a judgement in which he assumes himself as 'being Herbert'. Herbert can easily compose grammatically correct sentences, in which predicates and subjects are correctly manipulated, as long as *he* is not involved in any sense. Consider, for instance, the grammatically correct forms in the following protective discourse:

> One has to put on shoes before putting on trousers, because otherwise the trousers make blood. I can't eat red oranges or red cheese, only yellow cheese; I can't eat red grapes in winter, only black ones in summer, nor can I eat red currants or red apple sauce. (Sterba 1933: 35-36, my translation)

Yet how different these sentences become when they are related to his being, as matters concerning naming and judging *himself*.

I can only select a few of the many remarkable linguistic fragments in this case. For instance, Herbert says: 'Only living things have a name, things that live and that can be killed'. How remarkable that he grasps the fact that living things have a very peculiar status, that they are those things which have a special relation to names. He makes a similar point in an even more explicit way:

> One cannot just have name, one has to be someone, otherwise one cannot live. Therefore, I refuse to say my name, I shall only pronounce my name when I am someone. I want to be alive and grown-up. All adults have a name and are something. I *am* not the Herbert. Mama just says this; that is only my *name*, I know, I *am* really the wagon-manufacturer. (Sterba 1933: 17, my translation)

Even though Herbert does not succeed in progressing from the stage of having to that of being, it is quite remarkable that he can say so. He is able to say that he is not yet someone, but that he might become someone. It is as if he is longing to become someone. But how can one long for that which one is not, that which one does not have, or that of which one has no experience? This remains a mystery to me.

The clinical picture may be there, but the explanations remain very vague at the moment. Quite clearly, this is a problem for any theory concerned with the origins of intentionality.

Conclusion

'Only living things have a name, things that live and that can be killed'. In his own way, Herbert expresses how that which escapes understanding, that which cannot be retraced to memories of the body, and which—therefore—remains external, is likely to be 'a structured thing', something that 'stays together', and deserves to have a name. For him, such things have a risky existential status, because they can be killed. Herbert is mysteriously aware of this, because he cannot grasp his own structured being. This clearly is a problem related both to his material way of being in the world, and to the assumption of this being through language.

In my view, Herbert is an ideal illustration of the fact that structure is a forced move when one is interested in the origins of cognition. Firstly, because cognition is a matter of *systems*. Secondly, because, in order to study the origins of cognition, one must subscribe to the idea that what has happened has somehow left an inscription. These inscriptions might include: physical and bodily experiences (holes in the body, places associated with pleasure and unpleasure, the fact of observing differences between bodies) as well as experiences of language, of external objects, of mobility and immobility, and observation of things which are similar or dissimilar to us. All of these factors create the associative or logical pathways which ensure that the system 'stays together'; they also determine the paths along which future actions will be undertaken. If one recognises this historical viewpoint, a structuralist stance logically follows. Structure expresses the fact that, due to past experiences, not everything is possible. This is because history creates a space within which some things are viable and others are not.

Finally, structure is a forced move because human beings, as cognitive systems, are deeply involved with language. Evidently, human beings are organised, self-organising beings. They are also embodied beings, in the sense that they are in the world materially. But human beings are also developed in a universe of language. As Heidegger so aptly put it: 'human beings are promises, as well as slips of language' (Heidegger, 1959: 14). When Herbert says: 'Only living things can have a name', he expresses the central problem of cognition for human beings, even if this problem is not readily recognisable. It is the problem of how to *name*—that is, how to know these living things, how to know the fellow human being, how to know those that are existentially closest and dearest. Above all, it is the problem of how to find a place for oneself in the midst of similar beings and how to come into being as 'a slip of language'.

Becoming cognisant of oneself is unlikely to be a matter of building 'meta-representations'. If one takes a historical and basically interactionist stance when dealing with origins, one consequently changes the status of any 'meta-' or 'second order' construction. My conjecture is that grasping oneself through language is a matter of accepting an external description, which is locally and temporally adequate for internal dynamics, rather than building second order representations.

Notes

1 See, for instance, Marone (1999) on Freud's texts on hypnosis, and Dalto (1999) on the 'Project'.

2 I have translated all the passages from this case-study into English.

3 See Frege 1960; Dummett 1973, 1995; Kenny 1995; Le Gauffey 1991.

4 Frege adopts a triadic theory of meaning, in which a distinction is made between the sign, the sense and the referent. According to him, the sense-component has to be understood in objective terms: it is the means by which we determine the referent. In the case of nouns, the referent is the object to which the noun refers, and in the case of sentences it is the truth-value of the sentence. As an example: the nouns 'Morning Star' and the 'Evening Star' both have the same referent, namely the planet Venus, but they have a different sense—that is, there are, in this case, at least two ways to determine the referent. There has been much discussion about the status of the referent in Frege's works. Some interpret it along realist lines, others believe that an idealist interpretation is more adequate. For a discussion, see Dummett 1981; Sluga 1977; Tugendhat 1970.

5 Some might claim that Herbert's use of 'I' is not genuine, and that he does not really grasp the meaning of it. It is clear, however, that these genuine uses of 'I' pose a problem to this point of view. Likewise the statement that Herbert, being psychotic, is 'outside of language', clearly requires explanation.

6 I do not know what else call this; it is always difficult to talk about what is not. I also find it quite difficult to grasp the status of Herbert's refusal to verbalise the parts of his body.

FREUD'S PRE-ANALYTICAL WRITINGS AND HIS SCIENTIFIC REVOLUTION

Saul Haimovich

I present here a short summary of my research on the early, so-called 'pre-analytical' period of Freud's thinking. After a careful analysis of his writings, I have developed a model for understanding the changes that led him to a revolution in the field of human sciences. The essentials of his revolution, I argue, were elaborated in three major books: *The Interpretation of Dreams* (1900), *The Psychopathology of Everyday Life* (1901) and *Jokes and Their Relation to the Unconscious* (1905b). My research has led me to conclude that the theories developed in these works were the result of Freud's struggle to solve the problems raised by his early research.

Freud's theoretical development, in the years from 1883 until 1900, took place on two different levels that are only slightly connected. On the one hand, he developed a new treatment for the mentally ill. On the other, he attempted to develop a theoretical explanation of neuroses and psychoses and to elaborate a general scientific (that is, at this point, *neurological*) psychology to explain every psychological (normal and pathological) phenomenon. However, his failure to ground psychology in neurology—that is, his failure to transform psychology into a materialistic and naturalistic science—created an intolerable dilemma for him. According to his way of thinking (and that of his teachers and colleagues), psychology without a material basis was merely metaphysics, not science. In my view, Freud's new science was the result of his efforts to solve this problem (which I have termed 'the problem of the material basis of psychology') by discovering a *new* material basis for his ideas. This was achieved through an elaboration of the empirical aspects of his early inquiry into the stories told by his hysterical patients.

* * *

Freud's therapeutic evolution, from his adoption of Breuer's cathartic method until his treatment of Elisabeth von R., has been amply and kaleidoscopically examined by many authors. My central argument is that—in these first clinical cases—Freud's most important development was not his new therapeutic method, but his new empirical object of investigation—the life-story of the patient rather than his symptoms and illnesses. As Freud wrote:

> I was trained to employ local diagnoses and electro-prognosis, and it still strikes me myself as strange that the case histories I write should read like short stories and that, as one might say, they lack the serious stamp of science. I must console myself with the reflection that the nature of the subject is evidently responsible for this, rather than any preference of my own. (Breuer & Freud 1895: 160)

In these cases, then, we witness Freud moving away from investigating the origin and formation of symptoms, towards an ever deeper understanding of his patient's personal descriptions of their lives. It was these stories which Freud transformed into the central object of investigation.

Although this aspect of his work is very well known, my contention is that its function and meaning have not been fully appreciated by previous researchers. This development has crucial *epistemological* implications.

First and foremost the symptom lost its central importance, as the key means by which empirical facts are apprehended and interpreted. In Freud's new approach the symptom becomes an element *in a story* (and, for the most part, a relatively secondary, negligible element). As such, it can no longer serve as the basis of a system of classification, unless it is assigned completely different meanings to that which it possesses in the patient's story. This, of course, is a direct consequence of what Freud calls the 'over-determination of the symptom' (Breuer & Freud 1895: 173-4, 287-8). Alongside this we find other epistemological shifts in Freud's work, such as his conception of manifestly organic symptoms as 'psychic' in origin, and his rejection of any essential distinction between the normal and the abnormal. Freud's adoption of the patient's story as an empirical object of investigation led (as the quotation above suggests) to his estrangement from psychiatry. Although this epistemological shift is only implied in his earlier writings, it is developed explicitly in later works, such as *The Question of Lay Analysis* (1926). It should be noted, however, that Freud remained committed to both psychiatry and medicine, even whilst his own formulations led him away from psychiatry. The contradictions latent in his work, and the tension they caused, obstructed the full development of the new science he was creating.

Secondly, the study of Freud's changing empirical conceptions—that is, his way of perceiving his empirical objects of investigation—is a very fruitful topic of research. It was the gradual refinement of his analysis of his patients' stories, his adoption of the story as an empirical object, which provided the basis for his solution of the problem of the material basis of psychology.

* * *

The study of the problem of grounding psychology on a material basis rests on an analysis of Freud's first theoretical attempts to explain normal and pathological phenomena. These works include his first psychiatric papers on hysteria (1888d) and hypnosis (1888-89) and his monograph on aphasia (1953), followed by the theoretical papers accompanying his clinical research (1893c, 1894), and culminating in his huge theoretical effort to construct a general explanatory biological model of all psychology—the 'A Project for a Scientific Psychology' (1950).

Against the background of his new narrative apprehension of empirical facts, I analyse the psychological and psychopathological problems which confronted Freud at this time, focussing on his failed attempt to solve these in 1895. The study of these works shows that Freud's attempts to offer a psychodynamic explanation of psychiatric phenomena were only one aspect of a wider theoretical endeavour. His main theoretical ambition was to construct a comprehensive model of the psychic apparatus which would enable him to explain *every* normal and abnormal phenomenon of psychic functioning. This attempt, the 'Project' (1950), adopted the philosophical and scientific presumption that psychology was a natural science only if it were based on the German psychophysics and psychophysiology of that period. The 'Project' is Freud's attempt at an evolutionistic reduction of the psychoneuronal mechanisms, in order to solve diverse and complex physiological problems. Among these problems are: the existence and functioning of qualities; the reduction of language to psychophysiological explanations; and normal and pathological repression. The aim of this reduction was to explain the psychoneuronal functioning, and the phylogenetic and ontogenetic development of the psychoneuronal system as that which has to cope not only with external stimuli (as German psychophysics and psychophysiology asserted) but also with biological stimuli, originating from within the body itself. Moreover, Freud attempted to formulate this theoretical explanation within the framework of a materialistic and naturalistic ontology.

* * *

There are two traditionally opposed views on the nature of Freud's theories. On the one hand, biology-oriented interpreters claim that Freud's psychology is best understood when considered in its context of biological principles. Psychology-oriented critics, on the other hand, assert that Freud developed a psychology that came to be independent of biology. My approach differs from *both* these views by indicating the specific structure of Freud's thinking and by emphasising the profound dependence of all the elements of Freud's thought upon the psychophysical problem.

According to both traditional views, the most important issue is to decide whether Freud was essentially a psychologist or a biologist. I argue, however, that Freud's aspirations extended far beyond the desire to find the optimal distance between psychology and physiology (cf. Kris 1950: 115). In the first years of his involvement with psychiatry and psychology, he sought to solve the problem of mind-body dualism on a material basis. This was the central theoretical problem involved in all the various clinical phenomena which Freud investigated and attempted to explain at the time: hysteria, hypnosis, aphasia, and neurosis in general. It would seem that Freud chose these areas of study precisely because of their relation to the mind-body problem. For instance, when Freud moved from neurology to psychiatry he sought to explain how the brain produces psychological phenomena.

After his success in finding a psychophysiological formula for hysteria (Freud 1893c: 160-72) and in constructing an elegant nosographic architecture on the basis of the two elements (ideas and energies) of that formula, Freud felt he was now ready to undertake the enormous challenge of finding a solution to the most basic problems of the neurological explanation of psyche.

First and foremost he desired to find a biological (evolutionist and physiological) explanation to the riddle of *qualities*—that is, how consciousness emerges from physiological processes. Freud was confronted with this problem on several occasions—for instance, when constructing a psychophysiological scheme of sexuality (Masson 1985: 98-

105). Freud failed to solve this and other important problems in the 'Project'. These other problems included: the problem of 'backward discharge' as the explanation of hallucination and hallucinatory-like processes (Masson 1985: 160); why speech associations develop; and the localisation and functioning of memory—that is, how mnemic images are inscribed in the neuronal system. Freud stumbled over two general psychological problems. Firstly, he failed in his attempt to assemble two different models, one that could be called 'objectivistic' (to explain the reception and disposal of external energy) the other, 'subjectivistic' (to explain the work concerning endogenous energy). Secondly, he discovered that the great majority of psychological processes are unconscious (that is, *physiological*) and that consciousness is only a secondary and accidental feature of them. Almost all of these explicit acknowledgements of failure can be fully documented.

Freud's inability to find psychophysiological and evolutionist solutions to these problems in the 'Project' and subsequent works left him in a very grave dilemma. According to his presumptions, if psychology did not have a material basis, then psychology was not a science. However, at this point we encounter a most surprising development. It is as if Freud, failing in his efforts to reach the shores of Cathay, found himself on those of America. The failure of his psychobiological dream led him to create far more than a new psychology—in effect—a whole new science.

Though every Freud scholar is aware that Freud believed psychology without a material basis was not a natural science, no explanation has yet been offered as to what happened to Freud's reductionist dream after its collapse in 1895-1897. The approach I have outlined here allows us to fill in this lacuna in Freud's historiography. In my view, in place of neuropsychology, Freud constructed a new materialistic science, which could not be defined either as a part of biology, nor as a part of psychology. I will present some aspects of Freud's solution to the 'material basis' problem, and of his new science.

* * *

One of my main arguments is that in his reductionistic effort, Freud progressively moved towards an exact psychophysiological representation of linguistic phenomena. Beginning with the most elementary psychological phenomena—sensations, perceptions, memories—Freud attempted to use them to reconstruct and explain more complex linguistic phenomena. Influenced by Jackson's (1958) and Jerusalem's (1895) ideas on propositions and judgements, he reduced these to words, representations and propositions.

However, in *The Interpretation of Dreams*, Freud radically reversed this reductionistic approach. Instead of trying to arrive at a representation of linguistic phenomena starting from supposed elementary processes (obtained by a traditional de-constructive analysis of linguistic phenomena based on philosophical and psychological associationist models), Freud began his analysis of psychological phenomena through a direct appeal to linguistic phenomena, which he conceived as the empirical data of psychology. In other words, instead of trying to find the material basis of psychology in 'neurons', Freud now discovered an new empirical basis—the *text*—for a naturalistic and materialistic study of man. We might name Freud's new solution to the material grounding of psychology 'empirical materialism', in opposition to the 'theoretical materialism' of neurological reductionism. The latter is 'theoretical' because it uses neurons not as the empirical object of study, but as a purely *theoretical* device for explaining psychological phenomena.

With the establishment of linguistic phenomena as his object of research, Freud closed a very important phase in his intellectual life. I would describe this as Freud's 'pre-revolutionary' period, dominated by his struggle to solve the dualistic problem. At the end of this phase, Freud no longer needed neurons as a material basis for establishing psychology as a natural science. Linguistic phenomena—stories and texts—the new object of investigation, satisfied the demands of the 'hard sciences'; they constituted a material, observable, precise and objective phenomenon.

Inevitably, this development modified Freud's earlier understanding of the relations between language and thinking, and this had crucial implications. As we have seen, it was the linguistic text (and not propositions, judgements and representations) which was now the object of investigation. Consequently, it is no longer relevant to inquire whether Freud's theories are more 'psychological' than 'biological', or whether they retain any kind of 'biologism'. The important questions now pertain, instead, to the relation between the conception of empirical psychological phenomena (linguistic phenomena), and the adequacy of the psychological theories which Freud developed in order to explain these.

A comparison between these two different aspects—the empirical and the theoretical—shows that Freud's psychological theories, which are all based on the concept of 'representation' (*Vorstellung*), cannot fully explain the phenomena he investigated. Although Freud's new theories modified the traditional psychophysicalistic conception of representations (formerly regarded as a straightforward reflection of the external object), and re-cast the notion of 'reality' as dependent—instead—upon on *unconscious desires*, these theories were still based on a traditional, parallelist conception of the relation between thinking and language, in which the word receives its value from the representation (Ducrot 1968).

Contrary to his modifications, then, Freud continued to consider representations as the basic, elementary psychological units, and he based all his later theories on them. I would argue, in contrast, that representations, considered as units of psychological processes, cannot give a complete account of linguistic phenomena.

A review of Freud's different approaches to the relations between language and thinking has led me to the conclusion that his later, pure psychological theories (his so-called 'metapsychology') are no less reductive than his early psychophysiological theories. The new reductionism consists of a reduction of linguistic phenomena to representations (rather than neurons). I would describe this as 'psychological reductionism'. I would argue, then, that Freud's later theories must be considered in the light of the tension between two main tendencies: on the one hand, a conservative streak that caused Freud to remain loyal to old psychological theories; and on the other, a revolutionary urge, expressed especially in the various empirical and practical aspects of his researches. Freud was only partially successful in giving an adequate theoretical explanation of his empirical findings. The continued pressure to accomplish this hampered the full development of Freud's most progressive innovations. Freud's psychology acted as an obstacle to the development of the new science he had created.

* * *

Dream interpretation opened up a new world for Freud. He began to investigate a multitude of new empirical objects: errors, lapses, jokes, works of art, religious rituals and beliefs, cultural and social phenomena in general. His originality lies in his approach to these phenomena, which are not all linguistic. That is, linguistic phenomena were only the first stage and one part of Freud's empirical world.

The empirical objects of Freud's inquiries (aesthetic, religious, sociological, cultural) cannot be defined as 'psychological'. Even though Freud presented his analyses and explanations of sociological phenomena as psychological, his hypotheses are also *sociological*. I would argue that Freud's choice of the name '*psycho*-analysis' for his science is inaccurate; it is misleading with regard to its empirical domain, and the wide span of phenomena that Freud actually investigated.

In Freud's later works a new dichotomy supersedes and replaces the body-mind dualism that characterised his early works. Freud's engagement with dreams posed him with the difficult problem of people's relation to their linguistic environment, and—generally—the problem of social relationships as such. Despite his psychological reductionism, however, Freud successfully formulated sociological theories, such as the Oedipal organisation of the mind. However, more importantly, he evidently regarded the division of the study of humankind into two sciences as misleading. I would argue that, in elaborating his theories, whether of a more psychological or more sociological nature, Freud also endeavoured to deny the importance of this dichotomy (psychology versus sociology) as a useful conceptual model for the study of human phenomena. His concept of identification is one of the most important expressions of this attempt (for instance, see Freud 1921: 65-144).

I conclude with some questions: if we abolish the division between psychological and sociological phenomena, how are we going to define and classify human phenomena when trying to investigate them? Which are the criteria that will direct our choices, if we do not accept that there is an essential difference between psychological and sociological phenomena? My tentative answer, taking Freud as my lead, is that, firstly, the selection of human phenomena must be done on the basis of their phenomenological similarity (not of their social or psychic character) as in Freud's joint study of obsessive and religious acts (Freud 1907). Secondly, and perhaps more importantly, it is possible to explain the two kinds of phenomena as expressions of *similar unconscious desires*. It is my belief that these criteria could provide the basis for the development of a scientific study of man, and I present them as suggestions for future research.

THE ORIGIN OF THE SUBJECT FROM THE PERSPECTIVE OF FREUD'S SCIENTIFIC MATERIALISM[1]

Silvana Dalto

Introduction

It is undeniable that the subject emerges as a problem in the history of modern thought. This is what Wittgenstein summed up in the *Tractatus,* when he stated that the idea of the subject is metaphysical, as such unverifiable, and that it should therefore be left outside of science (Wittgenstein 1961: 5.631-5.641). This claim encapsulates the essence of a problem which begins with Descartes; after him, effectively, the subject which we must presuppose in scientific discourse is conceived of as something non-extended and transcendent—in other words, as something absolutely cut off from the human organism.

If such a presupposition, however, was indispensable in founding the absolute generality of the *cogito,* ie. the absolute sprit—in that it made the non-extended point into a constant, always self-identical reference for the fluctuations of knowledge, then on the other hand it also entailed that the subject, obliged to be the ethical response of the scientific endeavour, became—in a sense—impossible to locate. Once the subject has been founded in its transcendence and non-extension, every individual is no more than an irresponsible machine, filled with variable appetites of which nothing can be said with certainty (Baldini 1993: 61-72).

All this has had terrible consequences for the modern world, leading us into an increasingly rock-solid division between science and ethics. In my view, it is the abdication of science when confronted by the question of the subject which comprises the fundamental impasse. Once the subject had been separated from a body reduced to a *res extensa,* the scene was set for that extraordinary boom of organicism which we continue to witness today. Concerning the psyche, however, such a reductionist approach has left aside those aspects of research relating to everything in the nervous system which has to be understood in functional, and not merely in structural, terms.

Such is the problem posed by Freud at the outset, in the 'A Project for a Scientific Psychology': how to reconcile the structural conception of the nervous system, as something tending toward discharge, with the functional conception which takes into account somatic processes as cathectic processes. For Freud, it is not a question of flattening out the two conceptions into one another, but of articulating their incommensurability (Baldini 1994).[2] Moreover, the opening pages of the 'Project', in particular those concerning the experience of satisfaction, show how Freud tries to deduce from the biological facts of the prematuration of human birth and the baby's inability to perform the specific action, the seeds of a moral principle. Thus, the experience of satisfaction 'acquires a secondary function of the highest importance, that of *communication*, and the initial helplessness of the human being is the *primal source* of all *moral motives*' (Freud 1950: 318).

The aim of our enquiry is thus to trace the origin of the subject in Freud's work, on the basis of its material determination—in other words, on the basis of an organism which, due to the effect of the external world, ends up by producing a formation not identical, but equivalent, to itself, and which is a function of the external world. In fact, I think that we would never have needed to conceptualise anything as strange as the subject, if the human individual had not shown that it had such an ambiguous relation to its own satisfaction.

To account for this, we should note that Freud begins with the principle that the nervous substance not only reacts to the external world, but that it acts with it, in other words it seeks to position itself in the real, as Lacan clearly brought out in his reading of the 'Project' (Lacan 1986). Furthermore, Freud posits that what he terms the 'perceptual substance of the living being' is not normally placed in a position of cognitive self-awareness. The factor capable of showing it to itself is for Freud the constant stimulus, which implies that the organism can only recognise its unity by identifying with the latter. This implies the fact that when I say 'I', this does not only refer to my organic individuality, but conversely to that same organic individuality in so far as it is *strictly equivalent* to the perceptual mirror in which it sees itself.

All of this triggers off a 'natural' semiotic process which is that of the origin of the subject, as it has been outlined by F. Baldini in an article, *Corps et esprit dans le projet d'une anthropologie psychanalytique*, which I will follow here (Baldini 1990).

Freud begins with the living organism, which from birth is plunged into a real that only appears to it in the form of a stimulus. Now this stimulus occurs in a double mode: either as a momentary, transitory stimulus, to which the organism reacts with a reflex action; or as a constant, and therefore unceasing stimulus, which is not affected by reflex action. This latter kind of stimulus, then, demands something more complex from the organism, something to which the first pages of 'Instincts and Their Vicissitudes' bear witness (Freud 1915a). There, Freud says that the organism recognises itself in that which it cannot escape through reflex action. The Freudian argument is simple and inspired: everything which I am able to escape from directly is not me; whereas everything which I cannot escape from directly is me.[3] That which shows itself to me as a constant, I consider to be internal to me; this is the Freudian notion of how interiority originates. The formula is thus not *if it is interior, then it is constant*, but rather *if it is constant, then it is interior, it is I*. This is where the famous *Real Ich* comes from, the 'real I' which Freud situates at the origin of subjectivation.

In order to explicate all this, we must make a closer examination of the very idea of the body. A Freudian notion such as that of *Einverleibung*, 'incorporation', whose conceptual implication is that something will form one body with the organism, is a clear indication to us that the idea of the body is not entirely reducible to that of the living organism. Likewise, the phenomena of disturbance of bodily limits in the psychoses indicates that the organism alone is not sufficient to allow the intuitive sense of its own body. Every mammal, in its intra-uterine existence, is a corporeality which extends in cells which have the same chromosomal patrimony: the intra-uterine body is thus made up of a foetal *plus* a placental component.

During gestation the foetal part of the placenta—which also develops out of the fertilised egg, and which forms a distinct part of the new organism—is the most active part, because it is what guarantees feeding, and what prevents the overflowing of constant stimuli. It provides the foetus with an essentially stable, homeostatic condition. At this level, it is clear, the body is identical to the organism.

Now, birth entails a mutilation of the body defined in this way, due to the loss of the placental component which performed what we could describe as its *vital tasks*. It is obvious that the living being—if it wants to remain living—must make a monumental effort to reconstitute that homeostatic totality which is able to perform the vital tasks. The organism is not a *vital system* like the body; it is merely a *living system* that is unable by itself to perform the vital tasks.[4] It must therefore annex itself to a substitute for the placenta that is able to reconstitute it as a vital system, thus as a body.

As is clearly shown throughout ethological studies, the relation of the so-called 'territorial' animal to its own territory is exactly of this order[5]: it is a relation of incorporation, in the sense of the territory 'forming one body' with the organism which inhabits it. This is why the territorial animal reacts to the invasion of its territory in the same way as it reacts to a direct attack on its own organism. For the territory, by guaranteeing its food, reconstitutes the 'homeostatic adequacy' required by the *Not des Lebens* which, as we have said, makes up every vital system.

But this is not all, for the human being, in relation to other mammals, is characterised by a specific prematuration at birth. In mammals in general the loss of foetal connections and the rupture of the homeostatic equilibrium of intra-uterine life entails the breaking-in of constant stimuli, such as hunger and thirst, which are no longer filtered by the placenta. These stimuli are dealt with by the specific action, whose task it is to bring about the experience of satisfaction. Due to his prematuration, man does not have the same relation to the specific action as the animal, as the child cannot perform it from the outset. For a certain period of time, an adult will have to perform it for him.

I will not go into details about the ethical significance of such an experience; Lacan has already spoken of it at length. What I wish to emphasise, rather, is that it lies at the origin of a vital semiotic process. But why introduce a semiotic process here, where there seems to be nothing in question but the mechanical facts of feeding?

The problem is that all mammals need to reconstitute what they have lost at birth, and to link the organism to a somatic complement that forms one body with it (a territory, for example). This is why the body, as a vital system, is more extended than the organism as a living system. And it is also why an animal's territory is always intimately linked to it. The animal's demarcation behaviour leads us to think of its relation to the territory as a relation between an organism and a sign. Therefore, this is not a direct relation to an object, because the territory is constituted precisely by the set of signs which indicate that the object of satisfaction is located in a certain space. To be connected to the territory, then, is to be connected to the sign which the object is, and which is—of course—outside the organism, but nonetheless on the inside of the body. Effectively, if its territory disappears, the animal's life is in danger.

If to this extent things are well-arranged for animals, the specific prematuration of his birth makes everything more complicated for man. Since, in fact, he cannot perform the specific action from the outset, then when the excitation of hunger appears, with what can he identify? As it is precisely the element that would give him the feeling of perceiving himself in the experience which he comes to lack (I mean the specific action), in what else can he recognise himself, if not in that very excitation?

Let us follow the processes described by Freud in 'Instincts and Their Vicissitudes'. The first moment in the constitution of the subject consists in the establishment of a continuity between the organism and the external world. The child has to reconstitute its body as a vital system; if it did not do so, it would soon experience a loss of life. It must therefore incorporate hunger, the constant stimulus; it must annex a bit of this real which torments it. If, in effect, the real offers itself to us in the form of a stimulus, it is precisely a bit of the real which is incorporated by the perceptual substance. This amounts to an unquestionable advantage since, henceforth having hunger inside my body, I only have to avoid self-consumption to thus ensure that hunger has an object outside of my organism. But if animals only need act, for the human being the active path is blocked from the outset.

Only a passive path remains open to the human. On the basis of a certain number of repetitions of the *Befriedigungserlebnis* ('experience of satisfaction'), brought about by the adult, it is in a position to transform hunger into a solicitation. However, if, for the animal, the latter is a solicitation of the object, then for man it is structured as a solicitation of the other, of the adult. The human relation to the object is fundamentally indirect. In this way, certain stimuli will be privileged. On the basis of this experience, the first inscription takes place of the real which Freud calls *Wirchlichkeit*, material reality. Since satisfaction occurs in the mouth, the latter 'becomes the place where satisfaction is expected' (Baldini 1994: 18). But expected by whom? By the stimulus; in other words, by hunger. It is thus necessary for hunger to be displaced from the stomach, where it was before, to the mouth, where it can become a demand. It is in this adherence of hunger to a bit of the organism, this action, this identification, that the *Real Ich* is produced, as the first subject, as what we will call the true subject.

But the *Real Ich* has a transitory quality. It is here that the problematic relation to satisfaction characteristic of man comes into effect in all its particularity. The latter, in effect, effaces the first glimmers of the subject, the *Real Ich*, because, if it is radically his own hunger, then what remains of him when the hunger is satisfied? Satisfaction takes place, to be sure, but it is no longer anyone's satisfaction.

It is starting from this question that a second phase begins, that of the production of a fictional subject, able to embody the site where the organism will be able to recognise its own satisfaction. All the misunderstandings of philosophy regarding this, in Hegel especially, derive from the non-articulation of this point.

If the Real 'I' were a constant function moving between the stimulus and its traces, due to the reduction of the stimulus to zero, nothing would remain but the traces, the *Zeichen* or signs of perception—but for whom? The perceptual substance which recognised itself in the stimulus is not in a position to recognise itself in satisfaction. It is because of this that the nervous substance goes on to reproduce for itself the stimulus; it does so due to a recathexis, at a deeper level, of the zone of excitation (the mouth, to continue following our example). It is here that the drive is established. But the drive reveals its true nature here: firstly through the fact that it arises by detaching itself from the constant stimulus, and also through its smuggling in as real an excitation that is no longer. Secondly, since the drive is constituted in the absence of any stimulus, it has no possibility of real satisfaction. And thirdly—this is the key point for our argument—this process entails that the organism, which wishes to recognise itself even beyond satisfaction, makes the subject rise again from its ashes. Thus, a second level of reality is constructed. If *Wirchlichkeit* was posited as the inscription of the real, this new vital movement gives birth to *Psychische Realität*. This second reality is produced out of the first, but it is distinct from it due to the fact that while the first derives from the presence of the constant stimulus, the second derives precisely from its absence and from its substitution by an equivalent which is no longer real.

Thus the second function of the subject arises, that which Freud terms the *Lust Ich*, distinguished from the first function, the *Real Ich*, by the fact that while the latter originated in a conjunction with the real, the *Lust Ich* originates in a disjunction from the real, which thus becomes its fundamental concern.

This is why we are able to make a very clear distinction between satisfaction and enjoyment [*jouissance*]. Enjoyment is produced as a refusal of real satisfaction: it is clear that *Wunscherfüllung*, the satisfaction of the desire which characterises the *Lust Ich*, is very different from *Befriedigungserlebnis*, the experience of satisfaction characterising the *Real Ich*, because *Wunscherfüllung* can only be maintained by a process of cathexis, and not by the process of discharge which is a feature of *Befriedigungserlebnis*.

Here, we could refer to the dream of the 'beautiful butcher's wife', discussed by Freud in *The Interpretation of Dreams* (Freud 1900: 147-151).[6] The dream's protagonist is the very picture of satisfaction; she lacks nothing. Nonetheless she has a desire for caviar, although she has asked her husband not to give her any as a gift; for the husband would in fact do so immediately. Here, the woman, almost overflowing with satisfaction, will identify with the salmon which a friend of hers likes, the salmon which the friend cannot eat because to do so might make her less skinny, and thus more appealing to the dreamer's husband. Therefore the dream satisfies the desire that nobody should have any supper, that the friend should remain skinny. In this way, through an equation between salmon and caviar, the two women both remain hungry; they are both the salmon and the caviar that no-one's mouth can touch. But, we ask, with what has she supported this fictional hunger, this illusion of hunger, which brings about the return of the subject beyond even the real satisfaction that had effaced it? This is what we see represented here: there is an equivalent of the stimulus (the desire, the *Wunsch*), there is the salmon (what the butcher's wife in fact had for supper), but the mouth, for its part, is not there. It lies dormant, something represented in the dream by all the shops being closed, as it is Sunday: the hunger of the drive only emerges on the mouth's day off, we might say. In fact, if the hungry mouth were present, wide awake, it would immediately expose the fictional nature of the *Wunscherfüllung*.

The triumph of the *Lust Ich* which this dream represents lies in the fact that it asserts itself as *Lust Ich* (through an identification with the object) beyond the 'homeostatic principle which governs the organism, through evoking a hunger beyond any satisfaction' (Baldini 1994: 20).

I am unable to explore in detail the later developments in the subjectivation of satisfaction; it is clear that this phase of the *Lust Ich*, its self-assertion as the refusal of satisfaction, must itself also be transcended, in order that the subject can eventually posit its own satisfaction. This development is completely centred on the function of sublimation.[7]

Empirical subjectivity and transcendental subjectivity

I think I have thus clarified my initial proposition: namely, that there would be no sense in speaking of the subject if man did not have such an equivocal relation with his own satisfaction, if satisfaction was not so disappointing for human beings.

We have posited at the heart of this whole process the experience of satisfaction. What is fundamental is that satisfaction lies at the heart of all our thinking, which has—as Freud puts it in the 'Project': 'eminently practical sense'. He continues: 'it is the original interest in establishing the situation of satisfaction that has led, in the one case to *reproductive consideration* and in the other to *judging*, as a method of proceeding from the perceptual situation that is given in reality to the situation that is wished for' (Freud 1950: 332).

In all thinking activity, what is important for man is to attribute satisfaction to it, which is not something that occurs automatically. But precisely the fact that satisfaction should be refused at a certain point implies that the goal of our activities as well as our thoughts always remains marked by incompleteness.

If, because of neonatal prematuration, man comes to recognise himself more in the domain of the stimulus than in that of satisfaction, and if satisfaction, due to its reduction of the stimulus to zero, emerges as what effaces the subject, it follows that perceptual substance has to bring about the subjectivation of satisfaction. The unconscious, as such, begins with the latency of the real object, thus with a delay. This is why man is a being affected by nostalgia, because where he finds satisfaction he has no knowledge, and where he begins to know something about it, satisfaction is nothing but a memory. The more we continue with the labour of remembering, the more we perceive that it is not possible to reach anything originary, elementary; we can only approach asymptotically the thing of our mind. This is what we have indicated concerning the production of the drive (Freud 1915a).

Nevertheless, if the experience of satisfaction remains the model of practical thinking, and by extension of all thinking, the way in which we reconstruct the real object, by getting closer to continuity, is implicit in the psychical modalities of the recognition of satisfaction. There are experiences of satisfaction which Freud centres around a pleasure that appears too much or too little; there are thus different modalities of the functioning of secondary repression. Freud begins with these modalities, from an empirical point of view. This is where Freud reintroduces, in all its grandeur, the empirical subject. The territory on which he raises the edifice of metapsychology is always that of empirical subjectivity.

When we speak of the empirical subject, it is to oppose it to every form of metaphysics we know in the history of philosophy. Metaphysics works, in effect, because it accounts for a representation of our position in a certain reality. I can content myself with being merely a nothingness amongst the incarnations of matter (nihilism); or equally I can revel in the thought that the world exists because I will it to (voluntarism); or, again, think that I am all that exists and that the world is only my mirror (idealism), and so on (Popper 1969).

What Freud shows to be empty is the idea of an absolute spirit. Philosophers must certainly have noticed that the subject cannot be single, given that there is a plurality of metaphysicians, as we have shown. There are various ideas of the subject, which become the empirical field for a metapsychology, not simply of metaphysics, but of various kinds of metaphysics.[8] Metapsychology is the attempt to unify the field of phenomena, but its perspective is always practical before being theoretical.

There is thus no 'oneness' in the modalities of thought; there is no *cogito* as a transcendent, but an immanent *cogito*, completely implicated in the body that it was produced in order to exclude. It is on this basis that psychoanalysis offers itself as an ethical science, by immediately re-introducing a subject that is, before anything else, a body. But we should affirm that the subject in itself is unknowable: we never recover anything but fragments of it. We can never restore the subject to its complete state, firstly because the underlying somatic process would always be unknowable; and secondly because the subject does not exist as such, but only *in abstracto*. In reality, there are only empirical subjectivities.

With Freud, the idea of an absolute spirit collapses. Such an idea is sustained by my thinking what is in my thought to be identical to what is in yours and his. It is the fulfilment of the Aristotelean *logos*: there must be a collective substance, and it must be a single substance, in order to be sure that it is in fact the same and knows no variations. Thus the idea of a single subject, which was produced by the Cartesian unification of knowledge, collapses.

Ultimately, the subject's very relation to the real is just as problematic; effectively, the real only appears to the subject to vanish immediately. Yet nonetheless this real will have left behind that pulsation of the subject which is the *Real Ich*, whose effacement leaves nothing but the instance of the subject, as such unconscious—in other words, the *Es*. This real of the subject which vanishes in satisfaction must be reconstructed by us along the pathways of psychical reality. But we can never reconstruct more than part of it. This is what results in the exigency of the thing in itself.

Conclusion

I would like to conclude by considering Freud's materialist choice. It is because he has deduced the subject of the organism—of the organism's homeostasis across practical mental fluctuations—that we understand Freudian materialism as the deduction of the *cogito* from sensorial matter.

We have spoken above of materialism as if it were a kind of metaphysics. In what respect is Freudian materialism to be distinguished from other kinds of materialism? Ordinarily, materialism reduces the human individual to a bundle of sense-perceptions. *Nevertheless, it accepts the absolute generality of a kind of immediate cognitive self-consciousness in the organism.* In this, I think, lies the *metaphysical* choice of classical materialism.

Conversely, for Freud there is no immediate self-consciousness in relation to certain stimuli (those which are constant). In relation to the latter, there is a split between perception and consciousness, in which the unconscious is located. In our presentation, in order to shed light on the dynamic of the subject's constitution, we set out from the fact that the organism picks out certain constant stimuli and goes on to recognise itself in them (*Real Ich*). For greater clarity we started with those stimuli which always return to the same place: hunger in the stomach, thirst in the mouth. This explains why such stimuli are privileged.

However, if we consider the *An Outline of Psycho-Analysis* (1940), Freud's materialist perspective becomes clearer still. Let us begin with the notion of 'continuity'. For the perceptual substance, there is a continuity of the real—in other words, a continuity of stimuli. The living organism is always open to perceptions, but we are conscious of this continuity only fragmentarily: there is a dissymetry in perception, between that which I perceive which is continuous, and that of which I am conscious which is discontinuous. This dissymetry fractures the bi-univocity of the system *Pcs*. In the *Outline*, Freud will declare that the underlying somatic processes which are completely unconscious constitute the true, authentic psyche, and that the subject is nothing but a function of such processes, which on their own are unknowable

(Freud 1940). Hence the hypothesis of a thing-in-itself of which we can only ever reconstruct a part.

In this way, Freudian materialism is the same as empirical realism, the necessary presupposition of any hypothesis of a transcendental subject. The *cogito*, reduced to the non-extended, suffered its first collapse with Kant; it became necessary to introduce the hypothesis of a transcendental idealism. But the latter must be supported by a profound revision of the *cogito*—in other words, by a different idea of empirical subjectivity and its role in science.[9]

We can clearly see, then, the solution Freud brought to the aporias of Kantian transcendentalism: from the structural point of view, to speak of the transcendental subject is meaningless, because it does not exist as such, it has no noumenal reality. At this level, there are only empirical subjects, hence individuals. Conversely, from the functional point of view, we can in no way dispense with a transcendental aesthetic, without which to speak of psychical reality would possess—in the final analysis—no authentic meaning, because it would be impossible to posit the generality necessary to make of it a mental category.

Notes

[1] This paper was translated from French by Luke Thurston.

[2] For the epistemological questions implicit in this incommensurability, see Assoun 1981.

[3] For the elements of this argument in English translation, see Freud 1915a: 119.

[4] For a discussion of the difference between 'living system' and 'vital system' see Baldini 1990.

[5] See, among others, Lorenz 1963, and Eibl-Eibesfeldt 1984.

[6] [*Translator's note*: In the *Standard Edition*, this dream is referenced as 'Smoked salmon—supper of'.]

[7] For an exploration of the processes concerning the subjectivation of satisfaction, in particular as they relate to sublimation, see Baldini 1994.

[8] The same articulation is to be found in Paul-Laurent Assoun's book *Freud, la philosophie et les philosophes* (1995).

[9] On this question, see J. Petitot-Cocorda 1985. I am referring to the introduction by René Thom.

SUGGESTIONS FROM THE UNCONSCIOUS: FREUD, HYPNOSIS, AND THE MIND-BODY PROBLEM

Fulvio Marone

Introduction

The Freudian approach seems to depend on 'the progress of neurological, psychological and pathological knowledge' (Bercherie 1983: 242). Hereby, medical knowledge is at once the transcendental limit of psychoanalysis, and also the condition of its possibility. Indeed, Freud arrived at the threshold of the psychical unconscious by the rigour of his *neurological* reasoning.

I aim to illustrate this thesis by drawing on the debate concerning hypnosis, which animated medical circles—especially in France—on the eve of the twentieth century. The elements of this debate, as well as Freud's position within it, I have derived from a series of articles written by Freud in and around 1890 (Freud 1888-89, 1889, 1890, 1891, 1892-93).

Hypnosis

According to Forel's detailed examination of hypnotism—*Der Hypnotismus, seine Bedeutung und seine Handhabung*—as reviewed in Freud 1889, by the end of the 1880s there were three principal explanations of the mysterious phenomena of hypnosis. These were:

1) Anton Mesmer's theory of 'animal magnetism'. Mesmer worked in Paris during the second half of the eighteenth century, and borrowed the term 'magnetism' from the field of progressive physics in order to furnish a rational justification for phenomena that he was able to induce in subjects by force of will. He conjectured that hypnotic phenomena were the result of a subtle fluid which permeated the entire universe. Some individuals (so-called '*magnétiseurs*') were endowed with a higher concentration of this fluid, and thus were able to channel and transport it to subjects with a lower concentration, who were receptive and reactive to its influence. However, 'mesmerism' was soon rejected by the nineteenth century and its prevailing zeitgeist of scientific rationalism.

2) Charcot's 'spinal reflex' theory. Freud's teacher, the master of French neurology, interpreted hypnosis as a physiological alteration of the nervous system, provoked by a series of external *physical* stimuli and requiring a certain neurological predisposition on the part of the (hysterical) subject. This was the *somatic* view of hypnosis, mainly associated with the 'School of the Salpêtrière'.

3) The 'suggestion' theory of the 'School of Nancy' (comprising Liébault and his student Bernheim). To an extent, this idea was preceded by a contemporary of Mesmer, the Marquis of Puységur. This point of view identified a single source for all hypnotic phenomena—namely, the presence of an *idea*, aroused in the hypnotised patient from outside, but which the patient perceives as emerging spontaneously from within himself. According to this theory—the theory of suggestion—all hypnotic phenomena are *psychical* in origin.

Freud and hypnosis

Freud always remained closer to Charcot's views than to Bernheim's in the debate between the two schools. This was not only due to his personal affection for his old teacher, but also to the conceptual opacity of some of Bernheim's arguments. This was highlighted by Freud in the preface to his German translation of Bernheim's book, *De la suggestion et de ses applications thérapeutiques* (Freud 1888-89). In hindsight, however, one can see that the uniquely Freudian view of hypnosis originates from the encounter and mutual contamination between the Charcotian and Bernheimian interpretations.

Freud stressed that one could not deny Bernheim and the School of Nancy. He wrote:

> the achievement in stripping the manifestations of hypnotism of their strangeness by linking them up with familiar phenomena of normal psychological life and sleep... and in its bringing to light the psychological laws that apply to both classes of events. In this way the problem of hypnosis is carried over completely into the sphere of psychology. (Freud 1888-89: 75)

I find it remarkable that one hundred years later Freud's evaluation of Bernheim also applies perfectly to his own psychoanalytic work. At the time he wrote these lines, however, Freud's thinking was as yet far removed from his later areas of research.

Bernheim's merits are indisputable, yet the term 'suggestion' remains vague and ambiguous, despite its place as the keystone of the psychological theory of hypnosis. As Bernheim himself wrote: *'tout est dans la suggestion'*. According to him, 'suggestion' refers to a type of psychical influence which can be differentiated from other communications in that (as noted above) it appears to arouse in the patient an idea which is perceived not as originating from outside, but as arising spontaneously from within.

Direct suggestion can be defined as a direct effect of psychical ideas which the hypnotiser arouses in the patient. For instance, the hypnotiser declares: 'Your right arm is paralysed; you cannot move it', and the arm of the subject drops as if immovable. However, hypnotic phenomena sometimes occur under other conditions. For instance, Freud describes how 'Charcot gives the subject a light blow on his arm, or says to him: "Look at that hideous face! Hit out at it!"' (Freud 1888-89: 82). The patient hits out at an unseen object but then—in this case too—the arm drops, as if paralysed. Bernheim regards these kinds of effects as also resulting from 'suggestion', but refers to them as *indirect* suggestions. However, a psychological analysis—in these cases—does not elicit a picture as clear as that obtained in cases of direct suggestion. This is because the idea that the subject's arm is paralysed is evidently not the product of the hypnotiser's suggestion, and it does not seem possible to arouse or provoke such an idea in the patient's consciousness. Freud writes:

> In other words, it is a question in these cases not so much of suggestions as of stimulation to *autosuggestions*. And these, as anyone can see, contain an objective factor... [For instance:] Shutting the eyes leads to sleep because it is linked to the concept of sleep through being one of its most regular accompaniments: one portion of the manifestations of sleep suggests the other manifestations which go to make up the phenomenon as a whole. *This linking-up lies in the nature of the nervous system* and not in any arbitrary action by the physician; it cannot occur unless it is based upon changes in the excitability of the relevant portions of the brain, in the innervation of the vasomotor centres, etc., and it presents *alike a psychological and a physiological aspect*. (Freud 1888-89: 83-84, my italics)

This passage which—a century later—might seem somewhat obscure, actually revolves around the kernel of what would become the Freudian epistemological revolution. I shall try to bring out the full significance of this passage by placing it in context with some ideas regarding the mind/body problem.

The mind/body problem

The intuitive understanding of one's being seems to correspond with two apparently irreducible phenomenological modes. These were described by the ancient Greeks as 'ψυχη' ('psyche') and 'σωμα' ('soma'); by Christianity as the 'soul' and the 'flesh'; by Descartes as '*res cogitans et res extensa*'; and as 'mind' and 'body'—or 'mind' and 'brain'—by our own day and age. However, although at first sight these two realities appear to run in parallel with one another, the way in which one is identified in terms of its relation to the other is actually asymmetrical. Indeed, theoretically, the nervous system appears to be in a position to account for the *totality* of human phenomena (at least, according to our present state of knowledge in the immediate present and in the foreseeable future).

To take hypnosis as an example, *direct* suggestion can be interpreted as an occurrence stemming from consciousness (that is, as an idea suggested to the hypnotised subject) which is linked to a state of cerebral activity. *Indirect* suggestion, on the other hand, refers to a cerebral state which is not accompanied by a corresponding conscious occurrence. If psychological theories have no difficulty explaining autonomous psychical occurrences such as suggestion (because, theoretically, the parallel existence of an organic phenomenon leaves these occurrences unaffected), nevertheless they meet with great difficulties when having to explain occurrences which are not echoed in individual consciousness. This is because consciousness is not just an 'accident' for psychology. In fact, the specific domain of conscious is that which is *perceived*—not by the five senses (as it is for objective events) but rather by the 'inner eye'. In other words, consciousness is the domain of that which is perceived *subjectively*.

In traditional terms, 'the psychical' refers to one's individual *consciousness*. This definition became formally explicit in the Cartesian definition of thought, as: 'ea omnia, quatenus in nobis sunt, et in nobis fiunt, et in nobis eorum *conscientia est*' ['all these things—as they are present in us—originate also in us, and there is a consciousness of these things in us as well'.] Hence, where psychical phenomena are concerned, consciousness does not seem to constitute a *contingent* property, as it does for somatic events, but it is—instead a—*necessity*.

On the eve of the twentieth century, the term 'non-conscious psychical phenomena' betokened a lapse into an unbearable contradiction, or—indeed—the negation of the very premises (the very substance) of psychology. At that time, unconscious phenomena could not be termed 'psychological'; like all other mute occurrences in the organism, they had to be approached in *physiological* terms.

The unconscious

Freud complied with what one might call the 'Charcotian objection' to the psychological theory of hypnosis, but he was later to reinterpret it in a way which revealed itself as symptomatic of his approach. Indeed, the analyst-to-be wonders:

> How does this affect the antithesis between the psychical and the physiological phenomena of hypnosis? There was a meaning in it so long as by suggestion was understood a directly psychical influence exercised by the physician which forced any symptomatology it liked upon the hypnotised subject. But this meaning disappears as soon as it is realised that even suggestion only releases sets of manifestations which are based upon the functional peculiarities of the hypnotised nervous system, and that in hypnosis characteristics of the nervous system other than suggestibility make themselves felt as well. The question might still be asked whether all the phenomena of hypnosis must *somewhere* pass through the psychical sphere; in other words—for the question can have no other sense—whether the changes in excitability which occur in hypnosis invariably affect only the region of the cerebral cortex. *By putting the question in this other form we seem to have decided the answer to it.* There is no justification for making such a contrast as is here made between the cerebral cortex and the rest of the nervous system: it is improbable that so profound a functional change in the cerebral cortex could occur accompanied by significant changes in the excitability of the other parts of the brain. *We possess no criterion which enables us to distinguish exactly between a psychical process and a physiological one,* between an act occurring in the cerebral cortex and one occur-

> ring in the subcortical substance; for 'consciousness', whatever that may be, is not attached to every activity of the cerebral cortex, nor is it always attached in an equal degree to any particular one of its activities; it is not a thing which is bound up with any locality in the nervous system. It therefore seems to me that the question whether hypnosis exhibits psychical or physiological phenomena cannot be accepted... (Freud 1888-89: 84-5, my italics)

In this passage, Freud perceptibly—yet, it seems, shrewdly—loses control of the debate and the problem. To my mind, this bears witness to a latent polemic in Freud's writing, foretokening the confrontation that would occur in three year's time with the 'localisationist' neurophysiology of the age (the '*Hirnmythologie*' of Freud's former teacher, Meynert [Bercherie 1983: 152-4]).

In a very clear-cut fashion, Meynert's approach opposed the cortex (the locus of 'conscious psychical processes') to subcortical structures (the seat of purely 'physiological activities' devoid of psychical correlation). Although Freud refuses this exclusive dichotomy between physiological and psychical phenomena (from an *operational* perspective), nevertheless he does not abandon his 'scientific' ambition to find an organic parallel for psychical phenomena. Indeed, he adhered to this even in his very latest works. However, by fragmenting the atomic cerebral centres into a sequence of *relations*, he makes his return to 'wishful thinking' more practical. Freud's interpretation is akin to that of his colleague Exner, whose *Entwurf zu winer physiologischen Erklärung der psychischen Erscheinungen* (1894) was published only a year before Freud wrote his own 'Entwurf' (that is, the 'Project' [1950a]). Freud holds that the multiple connections between subcortical zones and the cerebral cortex enable Charcot's 'physiological' to have constant access to the cortex—and thus, by extension, to the *psychical*. What is more, Bernheim's notion of the 'psychical' is conveyed by Freud in Charcotian terms by awarding it an *organic* basis in the cerebral cortex, thereby shedding the biunivocal relation it retained with *consciousness*. By virtue of the multiple connections between cerebral structures, the psychical comprises a constant flow of *physiological* activities, which can be regarded as the 'non-conscious' side (or, at least, non-conscious 'in equal measure') of the psychical activity. Consequently, 'psychical activity' emerges as a *diffuse property* of the nervous system, whilst 'consciousness'—even if this, too, cannot be localised—surfaces as an intermittent cerebral *quality* of *variable intensity*.

Conclusion

In between the lines of this and other publications was born a plausible precursor of what was to become the most remarkable Freudian 'thing': *the psychical unconscious*. In its inchoate form it first took on the guise of Charcotian neurology, gradually achieving an autonomy which, in our century, is widely recognised. This idea, like so many after it, was born from a trait of the 'Freudian style'—that is, Freud's proclivity to pattern psycho-linguistic problems on shapes, models, and profiles more or less 'consciously' borrowed from the biological sciences.

FROM THE ASSOCIATIONIST UNCONSCIOUS TO THE UNCONSCIOUS STRUCTURED LIKE A LANGUAGE

Guy Trobas

Introduction

Although 1900 is generally given as the date of the 'beginning' of psychoanalysis, Freud had actually coined the term some years previously, after his discovery of the unconscious and his theorisation of it on the basis of the closely-related concepts of defence, resistance, and repression.

The debate on the 'starting-point' of psychoanalysis provides an ideal opportunity to question again the evidence for the Freudian discovery. As Lacan put it, this might encourage us to 'disengage from concepts that are being deadened by routine use the meaning that they regain both from a re-examination of their history and from a reflexion on their subjective foundations' (Lacan 1977a: 33). Indeed, this process represents a first step towards what Lacan called the 'return to Freud'.

It is from such a perspective that I will present my argument. As a main point of reference, I have chosen the unconscious. Although I will not try to pinpoint the precise moment at which one can fully ascribe to the unconscious the status of a 'concept', I will attempt to locate the initial moment of a turning-point or change of direction within the development of Freud's theory—in other words, the point at which his notion detaches itself from an associationist conception, and becomes strictly specific and analytical. This was achieved from the moment Freud took into account the structure of language.

The determination of the hysterical symptom by associative creation

This initial moment becomes manifest in the last pages of Chapter Two of *Studies on Hysteria* (Breuer & Freud 1895), entitled 'Case Histories', in which Freud, with a mixture of incredulity and extreme prudence, introduces new ideas on the formation of symptoms. These ideas relate to what he calls the determination of the (hysterical) symptom (Breuer & Freud 1895: 174-81)—that is, the difficulty of discovering the matter from which the symptom is composed or that which lends it its formal characteristic. He distinguishes this from the motive (or cause) of the symptom, and also from its mechanism. Concerning these issues, Freud elaborated a powerful and assured theory in *Studies*. These new ideas challenged his 'trauma' theory of the symptom, but without destabilising its overall structure.

Initially, Freud held that secondary traumatic incidents, or 'occasional causes', bring back memories of a primary traumatic incident. Due to the absence of an appropriate abreaction, this produces a predisposing fixation—that is, a sort of psychic isolate of bodily, behavioural or ideational representations linked to the traumatic situation, in which an excessive tension reigns. Because the subject is, as yet, unable to abreact appropriately, this re-evocation gives rise to both the repression of certain representations which are re-activated from the first trauma, and the symptomatic actualisation of a bodily, behavioural, or ideational representation associated with *either* the primary or secondary traumatic incidents, or even with other moments in the subject's history.

The question of the determination of the symptom can, therefore, be expressed as follows: Why is *one* representation chosen as the symptom of a trauma instead of *another*? And why does it have a *delayed* effect? Unless one thinks the unthinkable—namely, that only one representation, which imposes itself univocally, *can* be associated with the repressed representations—then one is forced to presume the existence of some *rule* which affects the selection from the chain of pathogenic associations, a rule which itself implies the fundamental mechanism of 'association', on which Freud's theory so heavily depends.

Hence, in the *Studies*, Freud elaborates a theory which I have described as being powerful, and which focuses *on the determination of the symptom by the creation of 'psychical associations'* (Breuer & Freud 1895: 153). This theory implies a fundamental principle, and is based on two associative mechanisms. Firstly, the principle, which makes its presence felt in the *Studies* is as follows: that nothing in the *content* (or 'concept' as Freud called it) of the symptomatically associated representation predetermines it—*a priori*—to be linked with the sexual content of the trauma. This stands to reason; in order to remain outside the realm of defence or repression the former should be—as Freud will have it in his *Interpretation of Dreams*—irrelevant with respect to the latter. This principle is obviously very broad, but the following two mechanisms narrow it down.

The first of these is what Freud calls a fortuitous coincidence. This entails that the hysterical symptoms (conversion or otherwise) are composed of representative material which *coincides* with the primary or secondary traumatic incidents—for instance, pains, behavioural patterns, perceptive elements which were heightened at the time of the incidents, or even thoughts which crossed the subject's mind during the incident. So, even though the aforementioned principle can encompass an infinite amount of representations, the criterion of concomitance locates a hypothetically finite group of possible symptomatic representations. However, it still cannot account for the fact that, within this group, only *one* representation will be powerful enough to represent the entire pathogenic group.

To a certain extent, the second mechanism which completes this selective determinism can explain this. But just what is this mechanism? In order for the pathogenic representation to find expression in the concomitant representation, the latter must also be linked with a painful affect—that is, with physical or moral *suffering*. Organic symptoms, unpleasant perceptions, and representations of a painful act or idea are all instances of this, and stand out in Freud's case material. Such representations are selectively symptomatised, because they already represent suffering, and thus can easily form an association with the psychical suffering linked with the trauma. This criterion is known as the 'signifying community' or the 'community by concept'.

Let us make two observations on this criterion. Firstly, a similarity in meaning is founded on the supposed universal representative value of *suffering* as an affect. This creates the link between the sexual representation of the trauma and the representation which is embodied in the symptom. In other words, if we view the associated representations as being signifiers of both the sexual signification and of a particular pain, then the affect of suffering which creates their 'signifying community' takes on the shape of a *common signified*. This is the essence of Freud's theory of the determination of the symptom, in which the signified prevails over the signifier in the associative articulation, and the universal prevails over the particular.

Secondly, this criterion for the selection of the representative matter of the symptom still leaves a margin of doubt concerning the choice of the symptomatic representation. Why is *one* physical or moral pain chosen over another, when—as Freud admits—*all* the pains in the subject's history are potential candidates?

A logical impasse

In the light of the above, one is brought to the conclusion that these mechanisms which—according to Freud—determine the series of pathogenic associations, must only exercise a *partial* control.

This shift in view is the result of adopting ideas from the school of thought which initiated Freud's original theory—namely, the empiricism of Hume, to which Freud was introduced during Brentano's lectures and, again, whilst translating the works of Mill. Indeed, in Freud's notion of 'fortuitous coincidence' we can discern Hume's first associationist rule, which explains the links between representations in terms of 'spatial concomitance' and 'temporal simultaneity'. Hume names this '*contiguity*' (Hume 1985: 57-8), a term which Freud borrows. Furthermore, in Freud's 'community by concept', one can recognise the second of Hume's three associationist rules—namely, the obscure force of the principle of resemblance (Hume 1985: 57-8), denoting the operation of the imagination, which picks out similarities against the background of the representations' basic difference from one another.

I will not elaborate on the logical vices of associationism, which has become a dominant ideology in psychology since the nineteenth century. However, I will mention certain consequences which this covert influence has on the subject, and on the unconscious, in Freud's notion of the 'determination of the symptom by associative creation'.

First of all, an associationist bias presupposes a symptom whose form is the result of a series of factors which can be objectified in psychic space or in the space of the signification. In other words, its form is the result of a logic which is *extrinsic* to the subject, and which is congruent (on the causal plane) with the idea of the real trauma. According to this conception, the material of the symptom is something which imposes itself on the subject, and not something which can be 'chosen' in any way. The subject of the associationist unconscious is, so to speak, more a *reactional* than an intentional subject.

In this sense, and since it can be objectified, the associationist subject can be integrated into a scientific discourse. For example, in *Studies on Hysteria* all that is repressed or is the object of defence or resistance is always a representation closely connected to a shock, a violent scene, an offensive encounter, a separation, a mourning grief , an insult... In short, it is connected with something which already has a traumatic value. In other words, the repression or resistance does not imply the realisation of *a desire to* repress or resist (which would presuppose an intentional subject) but rather an abreaction, which serves to discharge the tension produced by an external cause.

In associationism, the unconscious and conscious thought are structurally identical. Both are made up of primary elements, which are vague and devoid of reality, and to which associationist philosophy applies the term 'representation'. At the very most, Freud ascribes to these representations the status of a more or less constituted signification or meaning, whose verbalisation may be problematic. However, he never considers the fact that their organisation is similar in both its structure and materiality to *language*. This idealist conception of representation, still pervaded his notion of the unconscious when he wrote *Studies*. However, in this work we can already trace the origins of the turning-point which was to bring about a substantial rectification—even, indeed, the subversion—of this notion. This came about as a result of Freud's new theory on the logic of the series of pathogenic associations in the determination of the symptom.

The symbolical determination of the hysterical symptom

Towards the end of the second chapter of *Studies on Hysteria,* the point at which Freud introduces this new theory, it is evident that he is aware not only of its specificity but also of its radical originality, which is why he gives it a name straight away. It was probably in the middle of the year 1894 that he wrote the following on the subject of Elizabeth von R.'s symptoms:

> ...this abasia, at the stage of development at which I came across it, was to be equated not only with a functional paralysis based on psychical associations but also with one *based on symbolisation*. (Breuer & Freud 1895: 153, my italics)

However, what is more striking with regard to the originality and the conceptual limit of this theory, is the *style* in which Freud presents it. The dialectics of this style are much less confident than usual; its progression is marked by the uncertainty of how he should classify this new kind of determination ('causal' or 'adjunctive'?), by hesitations about its validity, by contradictions concerning its effect on certain symptoms, by the reduction of its clinical impact (dissociated hysteria, dreamlike states, low mental level, etc.), by his incredulity and even embarrassment as he touches on the comical and ridiculous aspect of this species of determination. All this shows also that, at a certain moment, Freud's *listening* also changes: he liberates himself from the metonymy of signification and turns his attention instead to the *metaphoric* powers of the signifier. All this is borne out at the very end of the chapter, by his theoretical reflection on the corporeal roots of the symbolism of language.

I do not have the space to trace in great detail the shift in Freud's ideas on these pages of the *Studies*, but I shall make some comments on the conclusions Freud draws in respect to his idea of 'symbolic determination'. In the very final case he discusses in Chapter Two of *Studies*, the case of Frau Cäcilie, Freud writes:

> She complained... of being troubled by a hallucination that her two doctors—Breuer and I—were hanging [*pendus*] on two trees next each other in the garden. The hallucination disappeared after the analysis had brought out the following explanation. The evening before, Breuer had refused to give her a drug she had asked for. She had then set her hopes on me but had found me equally hard-hearted. She was furious with us over this, and in her anger she thought to herself: 'There's nothing to choose between the two of them; one's the *pendant* [match] of the other'. (Breuer & Freud 1895: 181)

How are we to understand the symptomatic representation in the statement 'the one is indeed the *pendant* of the other'? It is clear that the image of the two doctors 'hanging' (*pendus*) from two trees in the garden is by no means a figurative representation determined by the actual meaning of this statement—or, more precisely, by its signified: *pendant* ('match'). Hence, no meaning community between this statement and its symptomatic representation imposes itself on the subject. On the contrary, here we are dealing with a *figurative* representation, which can only be the result of a decision or choice made by the subject concerning the signifier *pendant*. In this case, the determination of the symptom does not involve the univocal conversion of a signified which is said to be universal, but results instead from the effect of a *particular* signified which the subject has created on the basis of the polysemous signifier.

To elaborate upon this a little: the form of the hallucination which stems from the signified *pendu* ('hanged person') is not universally constructed by the signifier *pendant*, nor by the utterance in which it was used. Deriving *pendu* from *pendant* is an operation performed by the subject which transmutes the signifier, to the extent that it can be incorporated into the abstract universality of its linguistic approach, into a personal signifier of the subject. By interpreting the signifier, the subject makes it his own. It is precisely because this signifier (*pendant*) acquires a particular meaning from the forbidden signified (in other words, a signified in relation to the enunciation *beyond* the statement 'one's the *pendant* of the other'), that it is repressed. It therefore assumes the status of a signified in relation to the signifier *pendu* ('hanged person') which, symptomatically, is substituted for it. As is demonstrated by the analytic interpretation, *pendant* becomes the repressed signified of *pendu* ('hanged person') which assumes the status of a symptomatic signifier, and allows the breaking-through of the repressed.

Hence we find, within Freud's theory, the same definition of the symptom as that given by Lacan in his Rome Discourse: 'The symptom is... the signifier of a signified repressed from the consciousness of the subject' (Lacan 1977a: 69).

Conclusion

With this change in perspective, which allows the signifier to prevail over the signified, Freud surmounted the logical impasse of the associationist approach concerning the determination of the symptom—that is, the incapacity of this approach to account for the contingencies of an association within a field of possibilities. It was due to this impasse—which resulted from the exclusion of the subject—that the symptom, for Freud, previously had the function of representing a *real* trauma. Now, however, in Freud's theory of symbolical determination, the symptom acquires the function of representing the subject of the unconscious, to the extent that an unconscious intentionality is represented in the symptomatic signifier. By replacing the enigma of intentionality with a logical impasse, Freud re-situates the central issue of the cause (which was objectified in the associationist scheme) in the realm of the subject, thus opening up the domain of unconscious desire.

I would like to point out, in passing, that intentionality in respect to associationism was a novelty in Brentano's lectures, which later inspired Husserl, as he himself admitted.

With this new conception, the subject is no longer seen as a passive and reactionary 'translator', at the mercy of false associative evidence concerning the contiguity and the similarity of representations. The subject can no longer be absorbed into the objectifying discourse of science. It is now promoted to an interpretative, intentional subject, which *creates* meaning by deciding which signified is attributed to which signifier. At the time, Freud referred to the signifier as a 'verbal image' or a 'verbal representation'. This possibility of making a choice or decision, which is what allows the representation to be characterised by the subject, depends on the nature of the signifier whose fundamental yet equivocal power Freud first glimpsed. Of course, for the time being, he confined this treatment to subjects 'in states in which mental alteration goes deeper' (Breuer & Freud 1895: 181 n.1). However, within four years, he extended its scope to those clinical phenomena which Lacan categorised as the formations of the unconscious (Lacan 1998).

Freud's initial reservations or reticence, to which I alluded, reflect his surprise at the discovery that the signifier prevailed over the signified. This prevalence lies outside the framework of the associationist rules within which Freud first attempted to frame his ideas. In accordance with these rules, he elaborated the functioning of the unconscious on the basis of *illusions* of consciousness.

However, his reticence, as well as his scientistic prejudices, crumbled in the face of his stubborn insistence upon the clinical phenomena he encountered. In this way Freud made the first step towards a new conception of the 'associationist' rules which govern the unconscious—namely, the logic of the *signifier*. It was from 1895-96 that he began to conceive the notion of 'displacement' and its structure although, at this stage, he only apprehended it from the economical point of view. Soon afterwards, in 1898-99, he began to conceive the outlines of 'condensation'. These are the two concepts which heralded Freud's discovery of the unconscious, and which can only be attributed to himself... and to the structure of language.

BIBLIOGRAPHY

Abraham, K. (1907) 'The Experiencing of Sexual Traumas' in (1927) *Selected Papers on Psychoanalysis* tr. D. Bryan and A. Strachey, London: Hogarth.

Accardo, P. (1982) 'Freud on diplegia: commentary and translation', *American Journal of the Diseases of Childhood* 136: 452.

Allouch, J. (1984) *Lettre pour lettre, Transcrire, traduire, translittérer,* Toulouse: Eres.

Amacher, P. (1965) *Freud's Neurological Education and its Influence on Psychoanalytic Theory*, Madison, CT: International Universities Press.

Andersson, O. (1960) Letter to Kurt Eissler dated 29th August, Library of Congress.

Andersson, O. (1962a) Letter to Kurt Eissler dated 16th April, Library of Congress.

Andersson, O. (1962b) *Studies in the Prehistory of Psychoanalysis: The Etiology of Psychoneuroses and Some Related Themes in Sigmund Freud's Scientific Writings, 1886-1896*, Stockholm: Svenska Bokforlaget.

Andersson, O. (1979) 'A supplement to Freud's case history of "Frau Emmy von N." in *Studies on Hysteria* 1895', *Scandinavian Psychoanalytic Revue* 2: 5-16.

Andrews, G., & Solomon, D., eds. (1975) *The Coca Leaf and Cocaine Papers*, New York: Harcourt Brace Jovanovich.

Anonymous (1994) 'Editorial', *Journal of the Centre for Freudian Analysis and Research* 4.

Appignanesi, L., & Forrester, J. (1992) *Freud's Women*, London: Weidenfeld & Nicolson.

Assoun, P.-L. (1981) *Introduction à l'épistémologie freudienne,* Paris: Payot.

Assoun, P.-L. (1995) *Freud, la philosophie et les philosophes,* Paris: Presses Universitaires de France.

Baldini, F. (1990) 'Corpo e mente. Progetto di un'antropologia psicanalitica', *Théléma: la psicanalisi e i suoi intorni* 2.

Baldini, F. (1993) 'De Moïse à Pythagore, de Descartes à Freud', *Le Curieux-Courrier de la Bibliothèque de Recherche Freudienne et Lacanienne* 15-16: 61-72.

Baldini, F. (1994) 'Godimento e verità nella teoria freudiana dell'atto psichico', *Théléma: la psicanalisi e i suoi intorni* 5: 7-48.

Barclay, J. (1964) 'Franz Brentano and Sigmund Freud', *Journal of Existentialism* 5: 1-36.

Bateson, G. (1979) *Mind and Nature: A Necessary Unity*, New York: Bantam Books.

Bercherie, P. (1983) *Genèse des concepts freudiens*, Paris: Navarin.

Bernfeld, S. (1951) 'Sigmund Freud, M.D., 1882-85', *International Journal of Psycho-Analysis* 32: 204-217.

Bernfeld, S. (1953) 'Freud's studies on cocaine, 1884-1887', *Journal of the American Psychoanalytic Association* 1:581-613.

Binswanger, L. (1970) 'Freud et la constitution de la psychiatrie clinique', in *Discours: parcours et Freud*, Paris: Gallimard.

Bloom, H., & Trilling, L.L. (1973) *Romantic Poetry and Prose*, New York: Oxford University Press.

Bowen, M. (1992) 'Sigmund Freud as a translator', *Sigmund-Freud-Haus Bulletin*, 16, 2.

Brazier, M. (1959) 'The Historical Development of Neurophysiology', in *Handbook of Physiology: Section 1, Neurophysiology*, vol. 1., ed. J. Field, H. Magoun & H. & V. Hall, Washington: American Physiological Society.

Brentano, F. (1872-73) *Plan Für das Psychologiekolleg*, unpublished manuscript, catalogue number PS 62 in the possession of Dr. John C.M. Brentano, Highland Park, Illinois.

Brentano, F. (1973a) *Psychology from an Empirical Standpoint*, tr. A. Rancurello, D. Terrell & L. McAlister, London: Routledge & Kegan Paul (originally published 1874).

Brentano, F. (1956) *Die Lehre vom richtigen Urteil*, Bern: Francke.

Brentano, F. (1973b) *Psychologie vom empirischen Standpunkt*, Hamburg: Felix Meiner Verlag.

Brentano, F. (1980) *Vom Dasein Gottes*, Hamburg: Felix Meiner Verlag.

Breuer, J., & Freud, S. (1893) 'On the Psychical Mechanism of Hysterical Phenomena: Preliminary Communication', S.E. II: 1-17.

Breuer, J., & Freud, S. (1895) *Studies on Hysteria*, S.E. II.

Brun, R. (1936) 'Sigmund Freuds Leistungen auf dem Gebeit der organischen Neurologie', *Scweiz. Arch. Neurol.* 37: 200-207.

Buchler, J. (1955) *Philosophical Papers of Peirce*. New York: Dover Publications.

Buelens, J. (1971) *Sigmund Freud, kind van zijn tijd*, Meppel: Boom.

Burnham, J., & McGuire, W. (1983) *Jelliffe: American Psychoanalyst and Physician & his Correspondence with Sigmund Freud and C.G. Jung*, Chicago: University of Chicago Press.

Busse, G. (1993) 'Ein groß wilder Mann mit Cocain im Leib', *Psychologie heute* 20: 52-57.

Byck, R., ed. (1974) *Cocaine Papers*, New York: Stonehill.

Carpenter, W.B. (1874) *Principles of Mental Physiology*, London: King.

Charcot, J.-M. (1991 [1887]) *Clinical Lectures on the Diseases of the Nervous System*, tr. T. Savill, London: Routledge.

Charraud, N. (1997) *Lacan et les mathématiques*, Paris: Anthropos-Economica.

Chusid, J. (1985) *Correlative Neuroanatomy and Functional Neuroanatomy*, nineteenth edition, Los Altos CA: Lange Medical Publications.

Clastres, G. (1990) 'The Symptom', *Seminar of the Freudian Field in Israel*.

Dalbiez, R. (1941) *Psychoanalytical Method and the Doctrine of Freud*, vol. 2, London: Longmans, Green & Co.

Dalto, S. (1999) 'The Genesis of the Subject from the Perspective of Freudian Scientific Materialism', this volume.

Davidson, D. (1982) Paradoxes of Irrationality, in *Philosophical Essays on Freud*, ed. R. Wollheim & J. Hopkins, Cambridge: Cambridge University Press.

Deleuze, G. (1993) *Critique et clinique*, Paris: Les Éditions de Minuit.

Deleuze, G., & Guattari, F. (1991) *Qu'est-ce que la philosophie?*, Paris: Editions de Minuit.

Denzler, A. (1933) *Die Sulzer von Winterthur*, 2 vols., Winterthur.

Derrida, J. (1972) 'La pharmacie de Platon', in *La dissémination*, Paris: Editions du Seuil.

Ducrot, O. (1968) *Le structuralisme en Linguistique*, Paris: Editions du Seuil.

Dummett, M. (1973) *Frege, Philosophy of Language*, London: Duckworth.

Dummett, M. (1981) *The Interpretation of Frege's Philosophy*, London: Duckworth.

Dummett, M. (1995) *Origins of Analytical Philosophy*, London: Duckworth.

Edelman, G. (1991) *Bright Air, Brilliant Fire, On the Matter of the Mind*, New York: Basic Books.

Eibl-Eibesfeldt, I. (1984) *Die Biologie des menschlichen Verhaltens. Grundriss der Humanethologie*, München: R. Piper Gmbtt.

Eissler, K. (1964) 'Mankind at its best', *Journal of the American Psychoanalytic Association* 12: 187-222.

Eliot, T.S. (1963) 'East Coker', in *Collected Poems of T.S. Eliot*, London: Faber & Faber.

Ellenberger, H. (1970) *The Discovery of the Unconscious: The History and Evolution of Dynamic Psychiatry*, New York: Basic Books.

Ellenberger, H. (1977) 'L'historie d'Emmy von N.', *L'Evolution Psychiatrique* 42: 519-540.

Ellenberger, H. (1993) 'The Story "Emmy von N.": a Critical Study with New Documents', in *Beyond the Unconscious: Essays of Henri F. Ellenberger in the History of Psychiatry*, ed. M. Micale, Princeton NJ: Princeton University Press.

Engel, P. (1992) *États d'esprit: question de philosophie de l'esprit*, Aix-en Provence: Alinea.

Evans, D. (1996) *An Introductory Dictionary of Lacanian Psychoanalysis*, London & New York: Routledge.

Evrard, A. (1995) 'Wat Guislain reeds voorzag', *Tijdschrift voor Geneeskunde* 51, 7: 521-524.

Exner, S. (1894) *Entwurf zu einer physiologischen Erklärung der psychischen Erscheinungen*, Leipzig und Wenen: Franz Deuticke.

Eyguesier, P. (1983) *Comment Freud devint drogman. Étude sur la coca et la cocaïne à la Belle Époque*, Paris: Navarin.

Fink, B. (1995) 'Science and Psychoanalysis', in *Reading Seminar XI: Lacan's Four Fundamental Concepts of Psychoanalysis*, ed. R. Feldstein, B. Fink & J. Maire, Albany NY: State University of New York Press.

Flanagan, O. (1986) *The Science of the Mind*, Cambridge, MA: Bradford/MIT.

Flournoy, T. (1995) *From India to the Planet Mars: A Case of Multiple Personality with Imaginary Languages*, Princeton: Princeton University Press. (Originally published 1899.)

Fodor, J. (1982) 'Methodological Solipsism Considered as a Research Strategy in Cognitive Psychology', in Husserl, *Intentionality and Cognitive Science*, ed. H. Dreyfus, Cambridge AM: MIT Press, Bradford Books.

Forrester, J. (1980) *Language and the Origins of Psychoanalysis*, London: Macmillan.

Foucault, M. (1988) *Naissance de la clinique*, Paris: P.U.F.

Frampton, M. (1991) 'Considerations on the role of Brentano's concept of intentionality in Freud's repudiation of the seduction theory', *International Review of Psycho-Analysis* 18, 37: 57-83.

Frege, G. (1960) *Translations from the Philosophical Writings*, ed. P. Geach & M. Black, Basil Blackwell, Oxford.

Freud, S. (1877) 'Über den Ursprung der hinteren Nervenwurzeln im Rückenmarke von Ammocoetes (Petromyzon Planeri)', *Sitzungsber. Akad. Wiss. Wien* 75: 15-27.

Freud, S. (1878) 'Über Spinalganglien und Rückenmark des Petromyzon', *Sitzungsber. Akad. Wiss. Wien* 78: 81-167.

Freud, S. (1879) 'Notiz über eine Methode zur anatomischen Präparation des Nervensystems'. *Zbl. med. Wiss.* 17: 468.

Freud, S. (1882) 'Über den Bau der Nervenfasern und Nervenzellen beim Flußkrebs', *Sitzungsber. Akad. Wiss. Wien* 85: 9-46.

Freud, S. (1884a) 'Ein Fall von Hirnblutung mit indirekten basalen Herdsymptomen bei Scorbut', *Wien. med. Wschr.* 34: 244-246, 276-279.

Freud, S. (1884b) 'Über Coca' *Zbl. ges. Therap.*, 2: 289-314.

Freud, S. (1884c) 'Die Structur der Elemente des Nervensystems', *Jbb. Psychiatr. Neurol.* 5: 221-229.

Freud, S. (1884d) 'Cocaine' [in English], *Medical News* (Philadelphia) 45: 502.

Freud, S. (1884e) 'A New Histological Method for the Study of Nerve-Tracts in the Brain and Spinal Chord' [in English], *Brain* 7: 86-88.

Freud, S. (1885a) 'Gutachten über des Parke Cocain', in Gutt, 'Ueber die verschiedenen Cocain-Präparate und deren Wirkung', *Wiener Med. Press* 26: col. 1036.

Freud, S. (1885b) 'Beitrag zur Kenntniß der Cocawirkung', *Wien. med. Wschr.* 35: 129-133.

Freud, S. (1885c) 'Über die Allgemeinwirkung des Cocaïns', *Zschr. Therap.* 3: 49-51.

Freud, S. (1885d) 'Ein Fall von Muskelatrophie mit ausgebreiteten Sensibilitätsstörungen (Syringomyelie)',*Wien. med. Wschr.* 35: 389-392, 425-429.

Freud, S. (1885e) 'Zur Kenntniß der Olivenzwischenschicht', *Neurol. Zbl.* 4: 268-270.

Freud, S. (1886a) 'Akute multiple Neuritis der spinalen und Hirnnerven', *Wien. med. Wschr.* 36: 168-172.

Freud, S. (1886b) 'Über die Beziehung des Strickkörpers zum Hinterstrang und Hinterstrangskern, nebst Bemerkungen über zwei Felder der Oblongata' *Neurol. Zbl.* 5: 121-129.

Freud, S. (1886c) 'Über den Ursprung des N[ervus] acusticus', *Mschr. Ohrenhk.* 20: 245-251, 277-282.

Freud, S. (1886d) 'Observation of a Severe Case of Hemi-Anaesthesia in a Hysterical Male', S.E. 1: 23-31.

Freud, S. (1887) 'Bemerkungen uber Cocaïnsucht und Cocaïnfurcht mit Beziehung auf einen Vortrag W.A. Hammonds', *Wien. med. Wschr.*. 37: 929-932.

Freud, S. (1888a) 'Über Hemianopsie im frühesten Kindesalter', *Wien. med. Wschr.* 38: 1081-1086, 1116-1121.

Freud, S. (1888b) 'Aphasie', in Villaret, A., *Handwörterbuch der gesamten Medizin*, Bd. 1, Stuttgart 1888, S. 88-90.

Freud, S. (1888c) 'Gehirn. I. Anatomie des Gehirns', *Handwörterbuch der gesamten Medizin*, vol. 1, ed. A. Villaret, Stuttgart.

Freud, S. (1888d) 'Hysteria', S.E. I: 41-59.

Freud, S. (1888-89) 'Preface to the Translation of Bernheim's *Suggestion*', S.E. I: 71-85.

Freud, S. (1889) 'Review of August Forel's *Hypnotism*', S.E. I: 91-102.

Freud, S. (1890) 'Psychical (or Mental) Treatment', S.E. VII: 283-302.

Freud, S. (1891) 'Hypnosis', S.E. I: 105-114.

Freud, S. (1892-93) 'A Case of Successful Treatment by Hypnotism', S.E. I: 117-128.

Freud, S. (1892-94) 'Preface and Footnotes to the Translation of Charcot's *Tuesday Lectures*', S.E. I: 133-143.

Freud, S. (1893a) *Zur Kenntniß der cerebralen Diplegien des Kindesalters (im Anschluß an die Little'sche Krankheit)*, Vienna: Beiträge zur Kinderheilkunde.

Freud, S. (1893b) 'Über ein Symptom, das häufig die Enuresis nocturna der Kinder begleitet', *Neurol. Zbl.* 12: 735-737.

Freud, S. (1893c) 'Some Points for a Comparative Study of Organic and Hysterical Motor Paralyses', S.E. I: 160-172.

Freud, S. (1893d) 'Charcot', S.E. III: 11-23.

Freud, S. (1893e) 'On the Psychical Mechanism of Hysterical Phenomena', S.E. III: 25-39.

Freud, S. (1893-94) 'Accessoriuskrampf'; 'Accessoriuslähmung'; 'Agraphie'; 'Alalie'; 'Alexie'; 'Amnesie'; 'Anarthrie'; 'Anosmie'; 'Aphasie'; 'Aphrasie'; 'Bradylalie'; 'Bradyphrasie'; 'Dysgraphie'; 'Dyslalie'; 'Dyslexie'; 'Dysphrasie'; 'Echolalie'; 'Paraphrasie', in *Diagnostisches Lexikon für praktische Ärzte*, vols. 1 & 3, ed. A. Bum & M.T. Schnirer.

Freud, S. (1894) 'The Neuro-Psychoses of Defence', S.E. III: 45-61.

Freud, S. (1895) 'Review of *Die Migräne* by Paul Julius Möbius', in *Speciellen Pathologie und Therapie*, vol. 12, ed. H. Nothnagel, Alfred Hölder: Vienna.

Freud, S. (1896a) 'Heredity and the Aetiology of the Neuroses', S.E. III: 143-156.

Freud, S. (1896b) 'Further Remarks on the Neuro-Psychoses of Defence', S.E. III: 162-185.

Freud, S. (1896c) 'The Aetiology of Hysteria', S.E. III: 187-221.

Freud, S. (1897a) *Die infantile Cerebrallähmung*, in *Specielle Pathologie und Therapie*, vol. 9, ed. H. Nothnagel, Vienna.

Freud, S. (1897b) 'Abstracts of the Scientific Writings of Dr. Sigm. Freud (1877-1897)', S.E. III: 225-257.

Freud, S. (1900a) *The Interpretation of Dreams*, S.E. IV-V.

Freud, S. (1901) *The Psychopathology of Everyday Life*, S.E. VI.

Freud, S. (1904) 'Freud's Psycho-Analytic Procedure', S.E. VII: 253-254.

Freud, S. (1905a) 'On Psychotherapy', S.E. VII: 267-268.

Freud, S. (1905b) *Jokes and Their Relation to the Unconscious*, S.E. VIII.

Freud, S. (1905c) *Three Essays on the Theory of Sexuality*, S.E. VII: 123-231.

Freud, S. (1905d) 'Fragment of an Analysis of a Case of Hysteria', S.E. VII: 1-122.

Freud, S. (1906) 'My Views on the Part Played by Sexuality in the Aetiology of the Neuroses', S.E. VII: 271-279.

Freud, S. (1907) 'Obsessive Actions and Religious Practices', S.E. IX: 117-127.

Freud, S. (1911) 'Formulations on the Two Principles of Mental Functioning', S.E. XII: 218-226.

Freud, S. (1912) 'The Dynamics of Transference', S.E. XII: 97-108.

Freud, S. (1914) 'On the History of the Psycho-Analytic Movement', S.E. XIV: 7-66.

Freud, S. (1915a) 'Instincts and Their Vicissitudes', S.E. XIV: 109-140.

Freud, S. (1915b) 'The Unconscious', S.E. XIV: 161-215.

Freud, S. (1916-17) *Introductory Lectures on Psycho-Analysis*, S.E. XV-XVI.

Freud, S. (1921) *Group Psychology and the Analysis of the Ego*, S.E. XVIII: 65-143.

Freud, S. (1923) *The Ego and the Id*, S.E. XIX: 1-66.

Freud, S. (1925a) 'A Note Upon the "Mystic Writing Pad"', S.E. XIX: 225-232.

Freud, S. (1925b) *An Autobiographical Study*, S.E. XX: 7-70.

Freud, S. (1925c) 'Negation', S.E. XIX: 235-239.

Freud, S. (1926) *The Question of Lay Analysis*, S.E. XX: 183-258.

Freud, S. (1933) *New Introductory Lectures on Psycho-Analysis*, S.E. XXII: 136-157.

Freud, S. (1935a) Letter to Fanny Moser junior dated 13th July, Sigmund Freud Archives, Library of Congress.

Freud, S. (1935b) 'Postscript (1935) to *An Autobiographical Study*', S.E XX: 1-74.

Freud, S. (1937) 'Analysis Terminable and Interminable', S.E. XXIII: 216-253.

Freud, S. (1939) *Moses and Monotheism*, S.E. XXIII: 1-137.

Freud, S. (1940) *An Outline of Psycho-Analysis*, S.E. XXIII: 139-207.

Freud, S. (1940-41) 'Sketches for the "Preliminary Communication" of 1893', S.E. I: 145-154.

Freud, S. (1950) 'A Project for a Scientific Psychology', S.E. I: 281-397.

Freud, S. (1953) *On Aphasia: A Critical Study*, trans. E. Stengel, London: Imago.

Freud, S. (1956) 'Report on my Studies in Paris and Berlin, on a Travelling Bursary Granted from the University Jubilee Fund, 1886-6', S.E. I: 5-15.

Freud, S. (1960a) *Letters of Sigmund Freud 1873-1939*, ed. E.L. Freud, tr. T. Stern & J. Stern, London: Hogarth Press.

Freud, S. (1960b) *Briefe 1873-1939*, Frankfurt/Main: Fischer.

Freud, S. (1968) *Infantile Cerebral Paralysis*, Miami, FL: University of Miami Press.

Freud, S. (1989a) *Jugendbriefe an Eduard Silberstein 1871-1881*, Frankfurt am Main, Fischer.

Freud, S. (1989b) *The Letters of Sigmund Freud to Eduard Silberstein 1871-1887*, tr. A. Pomerans, ed. W. Boehlich, Cambridge Mass.: Belknap Press of Harvard University.

Freud, S. (1990) 'Gehirn', in *A Moment of Transition: Two Neuroscientific Articles by Sigmund Freud*, ed. M. Solms & M.A. Saling, London: Karnac. (Originally published 1888.)

Freud, S. (1992) *Zur Auffassung der Aphasien*, Frankfurt/Main: Fischer.

Freud, S., & Rie, O. (1891) *Klinische Studie über die halbseitige Cerebrallähmung der Kinder*, Vienna: Beiträge zur Kinderheilkunde.

Gay, P. (1988) *Freud: A Life for our Time*, London: J.M. Dent & Sons.

Geberovich, F. (1984) *Une douleur irresistible. Sur la toxicomanie et la pulsion de mort*, Paris: Inter-Editions.

Geerardyn, F. (1994) 'Aristoteles als "ik-ideaal": een lectuur van zijn droomtheorie', *Psychoanalytische Perspektieven* 25: 127-136.

Geerardyn, F., & Quackelbeen, J. (1996) 'Psychoanalysis and neuroscience: a particular *parcours*. Interview with Mark Leonard De Gier Solms', *The Letter* 7: 21-39.

Geerardyn, F., & Van de Vijver, G., eds. (1998) *Aux sources de la psychanalyse. Une analyse des premiers écrits de Freud (1877-1900)*, Paris: L'Harmattan.

Gomperz, H. (1936) *Theodor Gomperz. Briefe und Aufzeichnungen, Erster Bd. 1832-1868*, Vienna: Gerold & Co.

Grinspoon, L., & Bakalar, J.B. (1976) *Cocaine. A Drug and its Social Evolution*, New York: Basic Books.

Grünbaum, A. (1984) *The Foundations of Psychoanalysis: A Philosophical Critique*, Berkeley: University of California Press.

Haas, E. (1983) 'Freuds Kokainepisode und das Problem der Sucht', *Jb. Psychoanal.* 15: 171-228.

Hadamard, J. (1949) *The Psychology of Inventing in the Mathematical Field*, Princeton: Princeton University Press.

Hamilton, W. (1853) *Discussions on Philosophy and Literature, Education and University Reform, Chiefly from the Edinborough Review; corrected, vindicated, enlarged in notes and appendices*, second edition, London: Longman, Brown, Green & Longmans.

Heidegger, M. (1959) *Unterwegs zur Sprache*, Pfullingen: G. Neske.

Hendriks-Jansen, H. (1996) *Catching Ourselves in the Act*, Cambridge MA: The MIT Press.

Herzog, P. (1991) *Conscious and Unconscious: Freud's Dynamic Distinction Reconsidered*, Madison, CT: International Universities Press.

Hirschmüller, A. (1989) *The Life and Work of Josef Breuer: Physiology and Psychoanalysis*, New York: New York University Press.

Hirschmüller, A. (1991) *Freuds Begegnung mit der Psychiatrie*, Tübingen: Edition Diskord.

Hirschmüller, A. (1995a) 'Dynamometrie in 19. Jahrhundert', *Jahrbuch des Deutschen Medizinhistorischen Museums* 8: 97-102.

Hirschmüller, A. (1995b) 'E. Merck und das Kokain. Zu Sigmund Freuds Kokainstudien und ihren Beziehungen zu der Darmstädter Firma', *Gesnerus* 52: 116-132.

Hirschmüller, A. (1998) '"Inapte à être psychiatre?" La rencontre de Freud avec la psychiatrie clinique', in *Aux sources de la psychanalyse. Une analyse des premiers écrits de Freud (1877-1900)*, ed. F. Geerardyn & G. Van de Vijver, Paris & Montréal: L'Harmattan.

Holt, R. (1974) 'Drive or Wish?', in *Psychology vs. Metapsychology*, ed. M. Gill & P. Holzman, Madison, CT: International Universities Press.

Hume, D. (1962) *A Treatise of Human Nature: Book 1: Of the Understanding*, London & Glasgow, Fontana/Collins.

Hume, D. (1985) *A Treatise of Human Nature* [1739-40], London: Penguin.

Israëls, H. (1993) *Het geval Freud. 1. Scheppingsverhalen*, Amsterdam: Uitgeverij Bert Bakker.

Jackson, J.H. (1887) 'Remarks on Evolution and Dissolution of the Nervous System', in *Selected Writings of John Hughlings Jackson*, vol. 2, ed. J. Taylor, London: Hodder & Stoughton.
Jackson, J.H. (1958) *Selected Writings*, 2 vols., ed. J. Taylor, London: Staples Press.
James, W. (1950) *Principles of Psychology*, New York: Dover. (Originally published 1890.)
Jelliffe, S.E. (1937) 'Sigmund Freud as a neurologist: some notes on his earlier neurobiological and clinical studies', *Journal of Nervous and Mental Disease* 85: 696.
Jerusalem, W. (1895) *Die Urteilsfunction: Eine Psychologische und Erkenntniskritische Untersuchung*, Vienna & Leipzig: Wilhelm Braumüller.
Jones, E. (1953) *Sigmund Freud: Life and Work*, vol. 1, London: The Hogarth Press.
Jongerius, P. (1992) 'Review', *Tijdschrift voor Psychiatrie* 34, 2: 33-34.
Kahn, E.J. (1960) *The Big Drink: The Story of Coca-Cola*, second edition, New York: Random House.
Kaltenbeck, F. (1985) 'Sigmund Freud et Wilhelm Jerusalem', *Ornicar?* 32: 87-113.
Kant, I. (1986) *Critique of Pure Reason*, London: Macmillan.
Kant, I. (1982) *Critique of Pure Reason*, trans. W. Schwartz, Aalen: Scientia Verlag.
Kenny, A. (1995) *Frege*, London: Penguin Books.
Koestler, A. (1964) *The Act of Creation*, New York: Dell.
Kris, E. (1950) 'The Significance of Freud's Earliest Discoveries', *International Journal of Psycho-Analysis* 31: 108-116.
Kris, E. (1954) 'Introduction', in *The Origins of Psychoanalysis: Letters to Wilhelm Fliess*, New York: Basic Books.
Lacan, J. (1966) *Écrits*, Paris: Editions du Seuil.
Lacan, J. (1975) *De la psychose paranoïaque dans ses rapports avec la personnalité*, Paris: Editions du Seuil.
Lacan, J. (1977a) 'Function and field of speech and language', in *Écrits: A Selection*, trans. A. Sheridan, London: Tavistock.
Lacan, J. (1977b) 'The function and field of speech and language in psychoanalysis', in *Écrits: A Selection*, tr. A. Sheridan, London: Tavistock.
Lacan, J. (1979) *The Four Fundamental Concepts of Psychoanalysis*, tr. A. Sheridan, London: Penguin.

Lacan, J. (1981) *The Seminar, Book III, The Psychoses,* ed. J.-A. Miller, tr. Russell Grigg, New York: Norton.

Lacan, J. (1984) 'Compte rendu avec interpolations du Séminaire de l'Éthique', *Ornicar?* 28: 7-19.

Lacan, J. (1986) *Le Séminaire, Livre VII, L'éthique de la psychanalyse,* Paris: Seuil.

Lacan, J. (1988) *The Seminar—Book II: The Ego in Freud's Theory and in the Technique of Psychoanalysis,* ed. J.-A. Miller, trans. S. Tomaselli, Cambridge: Cambridge University Press.

Lacan, J. (1991) 'Metaphor of the Subject', trans. B. Fink, *Newsletter of the Freudian Field* 5.

Lacan, J. (1992) *The Seminar of Jacques Lacan—Book VII: The Ethics of Psychoanalysis, 1959-1960,* ed. J.-A. Miller, trans. D. Potter, New York: Norton.

Lacan, J. (1998) *Le Séminaire Livre V: Les formations de L'inconscient (1957-1958),* Paris: Seuil.

Le Gauffey, G. (1991) 'Frege l'exigeant', in *L'incomplétude du symbolique: de René Descartes à Jacques Lacan,* Paris: EPEL.

Le Poulichet, S. (1987) *Toxicomanies et Psychanalyse. Les Narcoses du desir,* Paris: Presses Universitaire de France.

Levin, K. (1978) *Freud's Early Psychology of the Neuroses: A Historical Perspective,* Brighton: Harvester Press.

Lewis, D. (1983) 'Anselm and Actuality', *Philosophical Papers* 1: 10-11.

Libbrecht, K., & Quackelbeen, J. (1995) 'On the early history of male hysteria and psychic trauma: Charcot's influence on Freudian thought', *Journal of the History of the Behavioural Sciences* 31, 4: 370-384.

Locke, J. (1689) *An Essay Concerning Human Understanding,* London & Glasgow, Fontana/Collins.

Lorenz, K. (1963) *Das sogenannte Böse: Zur Naturgeschichte der Agression,* Vienna: G. Borotha Schoeler Verlag.

Luce, G.G. (1971) *Biological Rhythms in Human and Animal Physiology,* New York: Dover Publications.

Lyons, W. (1986) *The Disappearance of Introspection,* Cambridge, MA: Bradford/MIT.

Macaulay, T.B. (1924) *Critical and Historical Essays,* vol. 1, London & Toronto: J.M. Dent & Sons.

Mackay, N. (1989) *Motivation and Explanation: An Essay on Freud's Philosophy of Science,* Madison, CT: International Universities Press.

Marcus, S. (1977) 'Introductory Essay', in *The Origins of Psychoanalysis, Letters to Wilhelm Fliess*, New York: Basis Books.

Mariani, A. (1895) *La coca et ses applications thérapeutiques*, Paris: Lecrosnier & Babé.

Marone, F. (1999) 'Suggestions from the Unconscious: Freud, Hypnosis, and the Mind-Body Problem', this volume.

Masson, J. (1984) *Freud: The Assault on Truth*, London: Faber & Faber.

Masson, J., ed. (1985) *The Complete Letters of Sigmund Freud to Wilhelm Fliess 1887-1904*, Cambridge, MA: Belknap Press of Harvard University.

Matsuno, K. (1998) 'Competence of Natural Language for Describing the Physical Origin of Life', in *Evolutionary Systems: Biological and Epistemological Perspectives on Self-organisation and Selection*, ed. G. Van de Vijver, S. Salthe & M. Delpos, Dordrecht: Kluwer Academic Publishers.

Matsuno, K., & Salthe, S.N. (1995) 'Global idealism/local materialism', *Biology and Philosophy* 10: 308-337.

Mauas, M. (1989) *The Seminar of the Freudian Movement in Israel.*

McAlister, L., ed. (1976) *The Philosophy of Brentano*, London: Duckworth.

McGrath, W. (1986) *Freud's Discovery of Psychoanalysis: The Politics of Hysteria*, Ithaca: Cornell University Press.

Merck, E. (1883-86) Archives, Geschäftsbuch.

Merland, P. (1949) 'Brentano and Freud—a sequel', *Journal of the History of Ideas* 10: 451.

Meyer-Palmedo, I., & Fichtner, G. (1989) *Freud-Bibliographie mit Werkkonkordanz*, Frankfurt/Main: Fischer Verlag.

Micale, M.S. (1994) 'Charcot and les névroses traumatiques: historical and scientific reflections', *Revue Neurologique* 150, 8-9: 498-505.

Mill, J.S. (1865) *An Examination of Sir William Hamilton's Philosophy and of the Principal Philosophical Questions Discussed in His Writings*, Toronto: University of Toronto Press.

Mill, J.S. (1879) 'Chapters on Socialism III', *Fortnightly Review* 25 (April).

Mill, J.S. (1880), *Vermischte Schriften III*, in *Collected Works*, vol. 12, ed. T. Gomperz, tr. S. Freud, Leipzig: Fues's Verlag.

Mill, J.S. (1889) *An Examination of Sir William Hamilton's Philosophy*, London and New York: Longman's, Green & Co.

Mill, J.S. (1971) *Autobiography*, ed. J. Stillinger, London & Oxford: Oxford University Press.

Mill, J.S. (1979), *Collected Works of J.S. Mill*, ed. J.M. Robson, Toronto: University of Toronto Press/Routledge & Kegan Paul.

Mill, J.S., & Mill, H.T. (1983) *Enfranchisement of Women & The Subjection of Women*, London: Virago.

Miller, J.-A. (1987) 'Neurosis, Psychosis and Perversion', in J. Lacan, *The Way to the Clinics*, ed. E. Pitchotka, Tel-Aviv: The Freudian Library.

Moser, F. (1925 [1901-3]) *Die Sinophoren der Siboyaexpedition*, Leiden: E.J. Brill.

Moser, F. (1935) *Okkultismus, Täuschungen und Tatsachen*, 2 Bd., Zürich: Orell Füssli.

Nassif, J. (1977) *Freud: L'inconscient sur les commencements de la psychanalyse*, Paris: Galilée.

Nassif, J. (n.d.) *Le projet de Freud*, unpublished seminar on Freud's 'A Project for a Scientific Psychology'.

Natsoulas, T. (1984) 'Freud and consciousness, I: intrinsic consciousness', *Psychoanalysis and Contemporary Thought* 7: 195-232.

Newell, A. (1980) 'Physical symbol systems', *Cognitive Science* 4: 135-183.

Nunberg, H. & Federn, E., eds. (1962-75) *Minutes of the Vienna Psycho-Analytic Society*, New York: International Universities Press.

Obersteiner, H. (1886) 'Die Morphiumsucht und ihre Behandlung', *Congrès périodique international des sciences médicales*, vol. 3, Copenhagen: C. Lange.

Panhuysen, G. (1990) *Het ei van Freud*, Amsterdam: Swets en Zeitlinger.

Petitot-Cocorda, J. (1985) *Morphogenèse du sens*, Paris: Presses Universitaires de France.

Petitot, J. (1990) 'Le physique, le morphologique, le symbolique: remarques sur la vision', *Revue de Synthèse* 4, 1-2: 139-183.

Pollak, P. (1884) '[Review of] Freud, Sigmund: Coca', *St Louis Med. and Surg. J.* 47: 502-505.

Popper, K. (1969) *Conjectures and Refutations*, London: Routledge & Kegan Paul.

Pribram, K. (1965) 'Freud's "Project": an Open, Biologically Based Model for Psychoanalysis', in N.S. Greenfield & W.C. Lewis (eds.) *Psychoanalysis and Current Biological Thought*, Madison & Milwaukee: University of Wisconsin Press.

Pribram, K., & Gill, M. (1976) *Freud's 'Project' Re-Assessed: Preface to Contemporary Cognitive Theory and Neuropsychology*, New York: Basic Books.

Ricoeur, P. (1970) *Freud and Philosophy: an Essay on Interpretation*, trans. D. Savage, New Haven & London, Yale University Press.

Riese, W. (1958) 'Freudian concepts of brain function and brain disease', *Journal of Nervous and Mental Disease*, 127: 287-307.

Rilke, R.M. (1988) *Selected Letters 1902-1936*, London: Quartet Books.

Rosenfield, I. (1988) *The Invention of Memory: A New View of the Brain*, New York: Basic Books.

Russell, B. (1961) *History of Western Philosophy*, London: Allen & Unwin.

Salthe, S.N. (1993) *Development and Evolution: Complexity and Change in Biology*, Cambridge MA: MIT Press.

Sauret, M.-J. (1993) *La psychologie clinique—Histoire et discours de l'intérêt de la psychanalyse*, Toulouse: Presses Universitaires du Mirail.

Saussure, F. de (1983) *Course in General Linguistics*, ed. C. Bally, A. Sechehaye & A. Riedlinger, trans. R. Harris, London: Duckworth.

Schib, K. (1970) 'Heinrich Mosers Briefwerk', *Schaffhauser Beiträge zur vaterländischen Geschichte* 47: 80.

Schott, H. (1981) '"Traumdeutung" und "Infantile Cerebrallähmung": Überlegungen zu Freuds Theoriebildung', *Psyche* 35: 97.

Schott, H.G. (1986), 'Freud's experiments on himself with cocaine as a forerunner of his self-analysis', *J. Ass. Int. Hist. Psychoanal.* 2: 7-9.

Searle, J. (1992) *The Rediscovery of the Mind*, London: Bradford/MIT.

Shapiro, F. (1989) 'Eye movement desensitisation: a new treatment for post-traumatic stress disorder', *Journal of Behaviour Therapy and Experimental Psychiatry* 20: 211-217.

Sheets-Johnstone, M. (1996) 'Consciousness', text presented at the International Workshop on Origins of Cognition, San Sebastian, 13-14 December.

Shepherd, G. (1991) *Foundations of the Neuron Doctrine*, Oxford: Oxford University Press.

Silverstein, B. (1985) 'Freud's psychology and its organic foundation: sexuality and mind-body interactionism', *The Psychoanalytic Review* 72: 203-228.

Silverstein, B. (1989) 'Freud's dualistic mind-body interactionism: implications for the development of his psychology', *Psychological Reports* 64: 1091-1097.

Sluga, H. (1977) 'Frege's alleged Realism', *Inquiry*, 20: 227-242.

Smith, B. (1994) *Austrian Philosophy: The Legacy of Franz Brentano*, Chicago & La Salle, Illinois: Open Court.

Soler, C. (1996) 'Time and Interpretation', in *Reading Seminars I and II*, ed. R. Feldstein et al., Albany NY: State University of New York Press.

Solms, M. (1996) 'Freud's solution to the mind/body problem', *Sartoniana* 9: 99-119.

Solms, M. & Saling, M. (1986) 'On psychoanalysis and neuroscience: Freud's attitude towards the localisationist tradition', *International Journal of Psycho-Analysis* 67: 397-416.

Solms, M., & Saling, M., eds. (1990) *A Moment of Transition: Two Neuroscientific Articles by Sigmund Freud*, London: Institute of Psycho-Analysis & Karnac Books.

Solomon, R. (1987) *From Hegel to Existentialism*, Oxford: Oxford University Press.

Sombart, N. (1987) *Nachdenken über Deutschland: Vom Historismus zur Psychoanalyse*, Munich: Piper.

Stengel, E. (1953) 'Introduction', in *On Aphasia: A Critical Study*, New York: International Universities Press.

Sterba, E. (1933) 'Ein abnormes Kind: aus seiner Krankengeschichte und Behandlung', *Zeitschrift für Psychoanalytische Pädagogik*, 7, 1: 5-38; 7, 2: 45-82.

Stevenson, R. L. (1885) [1994] *Dr Jekyll and Mr. Hyde*, London: Penguin.

Strachey, J. (1956) 'Introduction to "Observation of a Severe Case of Hemi-Anaesthesia in a Hysterical Male"', S.E. 1: 24.

Strachey, J. (1966) 'Editor's Introduction', to 'A Project for a Scientific Psychology', S.E. 1: 283-293.

Sulloway, F. (1979) *Freud: Biologist of the Mind: Beyond the Psychoanalytic Legend*, London: André Deutsch & Burnett Books.

Thornton, E.M. (1986) *The Freudian Fallacy*, London: Paladin Books.

Tögel, C., (1994) *Und gedenke die Wissenschaft auszubeuten. Sigmund Freuds Weg zur Psychoanalyse*, Tübinge: Edition Diskord.

Triarho, L., & del Cerro, M. (1985) 'Freud's contribution to neuroanatomy', *Archives of Neurology*, 42: 282.

Trobas, G. (1999) 'From the Associationist Unconscious to the Unconscious Structured Like a Language', this volume.

Tugendhat, E. (1970) 'The meaning of '*Bedeutung*' in Frege', *Analysis*, 30: 177-189.

Van de Vijver, G. (1996a) '"Who is galloping at a narrow path?": Conversation with Heinz Van Foerster 02/06/1995', *Contemporary Philosophy* 24, 11: 329-338 (in Japanese).

Van de Vijver, G. (1996b) 'Internalism versus externalism: a matter of choice?', *Contemporary Philosophy* 24, 11: 93-101 (in Japanese).

Van de Vijver, G., & Geerardyn F., (1992a) 'Introduction', in S. Freud, *Ontwerp van een natuurwetenschappelijke psychologie'*, trans. G. Van de Vijver and F. Geerardyn, Gent: Idesça.

Van de Vijver, G., & Geerardyn, F. (1992b) 'Over het statuut van het Ontwerp als psychoanalytische tekst. Inleiding', in *Het ontwerp—Sigmund Freud,* ed. G. Van de Vijver, & F. Geerardyn, Gent: Idesça.

Van de Vijver, G., & Geerardyn, F., eds. (1995) *Freud's Pre-Analytical Writings (1877-1900),* Gent: Universiteit Gent.

Van Hoorde, H. (1992) *Psychiatrie en psychoanalyse: scheiding van tafel en bank?*, Gent: Idesça.

Van Hoorde, H. (1993) 'Freuds "Ontwerp" of de omweg recht op het doel af', *Tijdschrift voor Psychiatrie* 35: 215-218.

Vera Ocampo, E. (1989) *L envers de la toxicomanie, Un ideal d'indépendance,* Paris: Editions Denoel.

Verbeek, E. (1971) *Geloof en ongeloof bij Sigmund Freud,* Nijkerk: G.F. Callenbach.

Verbeek, E. (1973) *De man met de glazen hoed,* Nijkerk: G.F. Callenbach.

Vom Scheidt, J. (1973a) 'Sigmund Freud und das Kokain', *Psyche* 27: 385-430.

Vom Scheidt, J. (1973b) *Freud und das Kokain. Die Selbstversuche Freuds als Anstoß zur 'Traumdeutung',* München: Kindler (Geist und Psyche).

Wallace, E. (1992) 'Freud and the Mind-Body Problem', in *Freud and the History of Psychoanalysis,* ed. T. Gelfand & J. Kerr, Hillsdale, NJ: The Analytic Press.

Watson, A. (1958) 'Freud the translator: some contacts with philosophy', *International Journal of Psycho-Analysis,* 39.

Whyte, L. (1978) *The Unconscious Before Freud,* London: Julian Friedmann.

Wittgenstein, L. (1961) *Tractatus logico-philosophicus,* London: Routledge & Kegan Paul.

Young, R. (1970) *Mind, Brain and Adaptation in the Nineteenth Century,* Oxford: Oxford University Press.

INDEX

For Product Safety Concerns and Information please contact our EU representative GPSR@taylorandfrancis.com
Taylor & Francis Verlag GmbH, Kaufingerstraße 24, 80331 München, Germany

www.ingramcontent.com/pod-product-compliance
Ingram Content Group UK Ltd.
Pitfield, Milton Keynes, MK11 3LW, UK
UKHW022001180926
475701UK00003B/137

* 9 7 8 1 8 5 5 7 5 2 8 5 6 *